FOOD
— IS A —
LOVE LANGUAGE

Copyright © 2022 by EAGLE EYE PUBLISHING GROUP

All rights reserved. This book or any portion thereof
may not be reproduced or used in any manner whatsoever
Without the express written permission of the publisher
Except for the use of brief quotations in a book review.

Printed in the United States of America

Identifiers: ISBN 9798987223307

Library of Congress Control Number: 2022921853

Creative Direction: Eimi El

Cover Photo: Juan Benavides

Food Photography: Juan Benavides

Published by Eagle Eye Publishing Group

Book Cover Design: James_ghdesign

Editor: James_ghdesign

Food Stylist: Eimi El & Juan Benavides

First Printing: 2022

FORWARD

Food is a love language that needs to be included in the conversation and I am happy to be the first to acknowledge it. Food brings people together for weddings, birthdays, milestones, showers, etc. There is something special about delicious food cooked with a whole lot of love, soul, and magic. I've been told by several clients "I can taste the love in the food." I take pride in this. When you talk about love, don't forget to mention food! Love is the highest vibrating frequency. To taste love through food is the next level of InnerG.

For some, food is emotional and for others, it's a normal lifestyle. I remember when I experienced depression, I would not have an appetite and food would taste disgusting because my InnerG. was low vibrating. On the other hand, I have friends and family who are the complete opposite. When depressed, they indulge in all kinds of cookies, fried foods, etc. Have you ever thought about your emotional connection to food? Food fuels your body with either high or low InnerG. I know we can all remember any dinner event, i.e., family gathering, cookout, party, the food is scrumptious, you eat multiple plates, and allow the food to digest. Then take a nap because you are tired, get up, have dessert, and now you are tired again! I know I am not the only one! Understanding your connection to food and how it affects your body will allow you to make better lifestyle choices.

When you analyze what you eat and why, it becomes easier to remove foods that no longer serve your temple. "Let food be thy medicine," Hippocrates. Food is created to heal your body on all levels. In no way should your body experience any trauma while or after eating. Eating whole food plant-based guarantees you will receive all the nutrients in its natural state. Your body is literally an InnerG and water field. The human body is made up of 45%–75% water (Cessions, May 2020). Over 200 vegetables contain high water content. Just as plants require water to grow, your body needs water to thrive, function efficiently and regenerate new cells.

I always had a love and appreciation for food and cooking. When I ponder the things I love, food is the first thing that comes to mind! I have witnessed people hum, dance, and sing while eating. Food makes you happy, relates to sentimental memories, and new experiences. Important announcements, surprises, or proposals are typically made over dinner. Food and love are synonymous with one another. When eating, consider food that loves you, hydrates you, and gives you InnerG.. No matter what you do in life, love your temple, you will only get one. Feed it with love.

I trust the recipes in this book and the love you feel when creating these dishes will inspire you to evaluate how you connect with food and why you love some of the foods you consume.

Thank you to everyone who encouraged, requested, and supported this project. It is one of my favorites. The goal is to give love, show love, and in all things, be love

With Love,

Chef Eimi Eagle Eye El

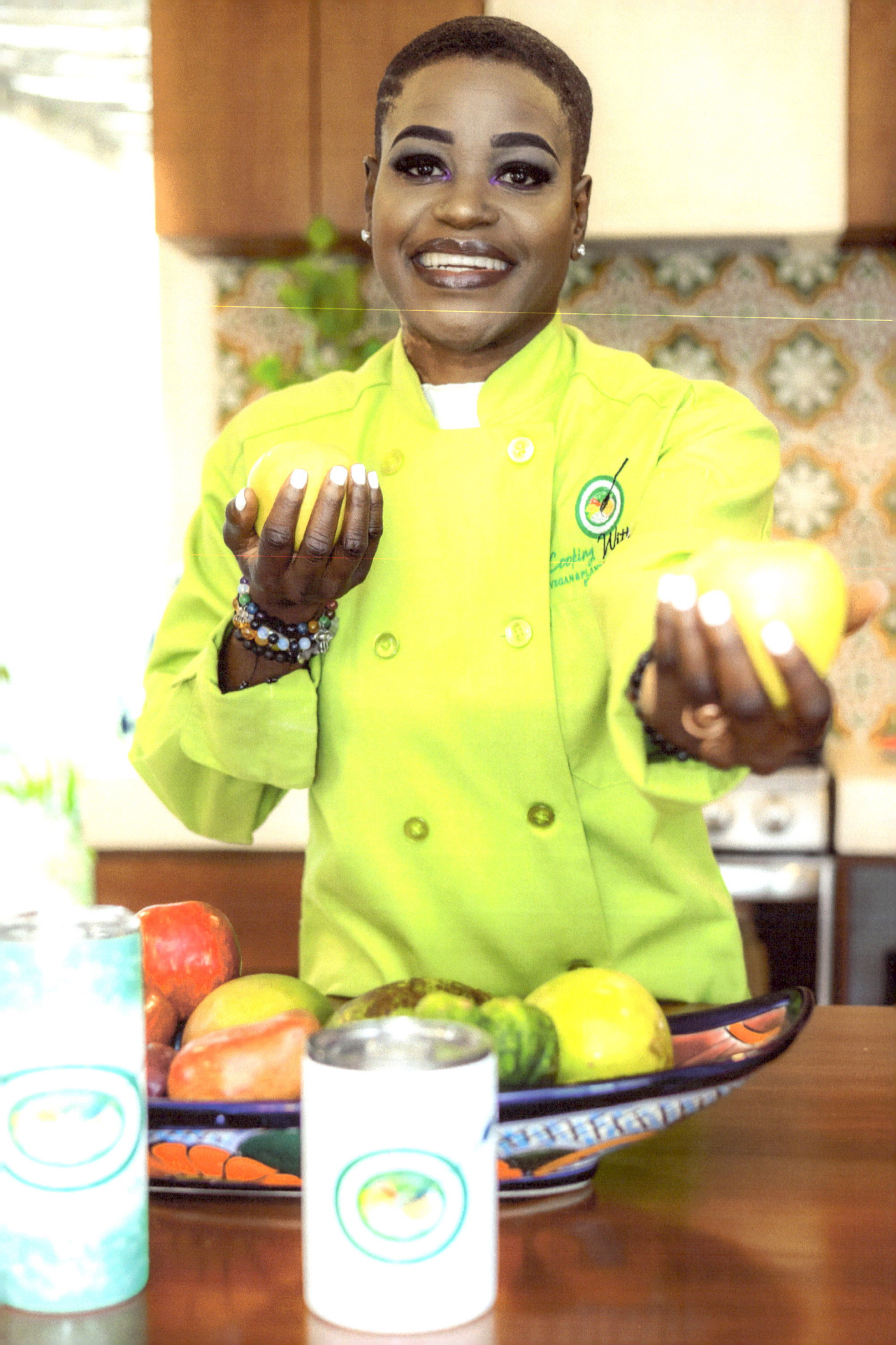

INTRODUCTION

"Food Is a Love Language" is a cookbook compiled of recipes for any occasion. I have prepared these dishes at family gatherings, celebrations, etc. I've even cooked most of them just because I was in the mood for good food. It does not have to be a special occasion or a celebration to prepare good food. Whenever you crave some good food get in the kitchen and start whipping, be sure to tag us when you do!

When I am preparing food, I know my ancestors are with me guiding me. I do not measure unless it's a new recipe or baking. Cooking is like a meditative form of art. I get in a groove and listening to my inner spirit and the rest is a masterpiece. **Please note: the measurements are not exact, allow your ancestors to guide you. If you are misguided, please meditate. Trust me, it works.**

As my connection to food matured, I realized that the love I felt was different but the same love as anything else I indulge in. I begin to ponder my love languages and quicky realized food is at the top of the list. Food Is a Love Language! Whenever I think of food, I get happy and sometimes even dance. I've witnessed people eat my food and make all kinds of noises, dance, and acknowledge the love. The food you eat has a tremendous effect on your mind, body, and soul. Consider your thoughts and mood when you're shopping for food, keep a journal of what you eat and how you feel, then implement small changes. The recipes in this book are inspired by my favorite dishes I prepare for family gatherings or celebrations. Food Is a Love Language is inspired by my love for food and passion of cooking for others and observing reactions.

CONNECT WITH US

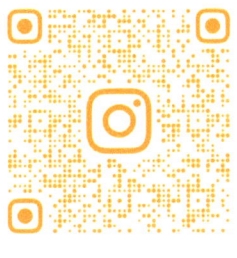

 info@eimielwellness.com

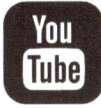 COOKING WITH EIM

CONTENTS

FORWARD 3

INTRODUCTION 5

MAIN DISHES 8–9

    BARBECUE NIBS 11

    MEETLOAF 13

    PAN SEARED OYSTERMUSHROOMS 15

    FRIED OYSTER MUSHROOMS 17

    JACK FRUIT POTROAST 19

    BARBECUE JACKFRUIT 21

    ROASTED CAULIFLOWER 23

SIDE DISHES 24–25

    CANDIED BUTTERNUT SQUASH 27

    COLLARDS 29

    CORNBREAD 31

    SAUTEED PURPLE CABBAGE 33

    CRANBERRY SAUCE 35

    QUINOA 37

    MASHED RED POTATOES 39

    BALSAMIC GLAZED BRUSSEL SPROUTS 41

    MAC 'N CHEEZE 43

    GREEN BEANS 45

    BLACK RICE 47

    POTATO SALAD 49

DESSERTS   **51**
    LEMON BUNDT CAKE   53
    CHOCOLATE COVERED DATES   55
    CANDIED PECAN MAPLE SYRUP DONUTS   57
    APPLE PIE EGGROLLS   59
    PECAN CHOCOLATE CHIP COOKIES   60
    SUNFLOWER SEED BUTTER COOKIES   61
    CANDIED BUTTERNUT SQUASH PIE   63

BEVERAGES   **65**
    SORREL TEA   67
    HOT COCOA   69
    STRAWBERRY LIMEADE   70

BONUS   **73**
    PHISH   77
    SCALLOPS   79
    JOYCE KRAB CAKES   81
    CALAMARI   83
    CHICKPEA SALAD   84
    SKRIMP   85
    INDEX   86-87
    BIBLIOGRAPHY   88

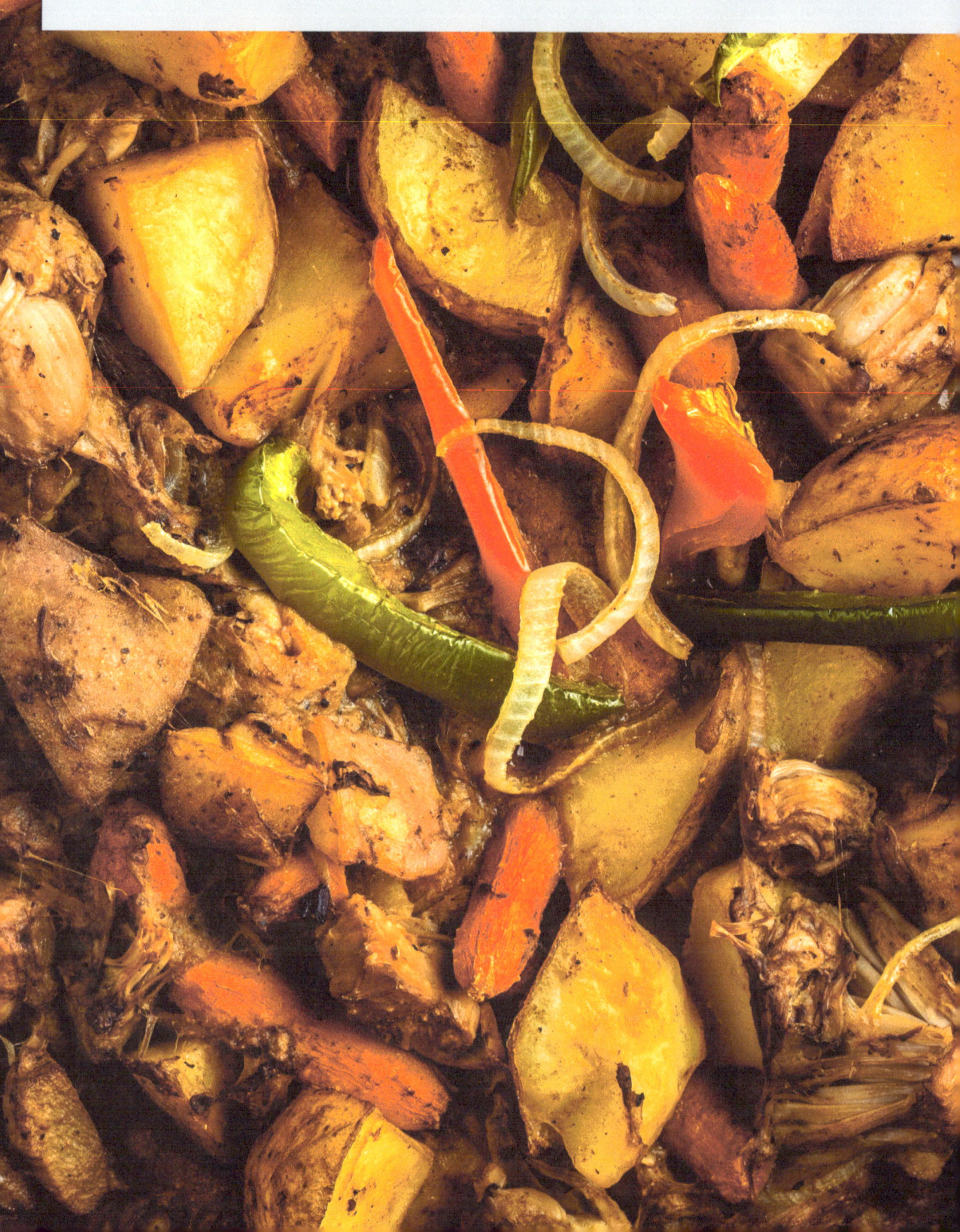

MAIN

DISHES

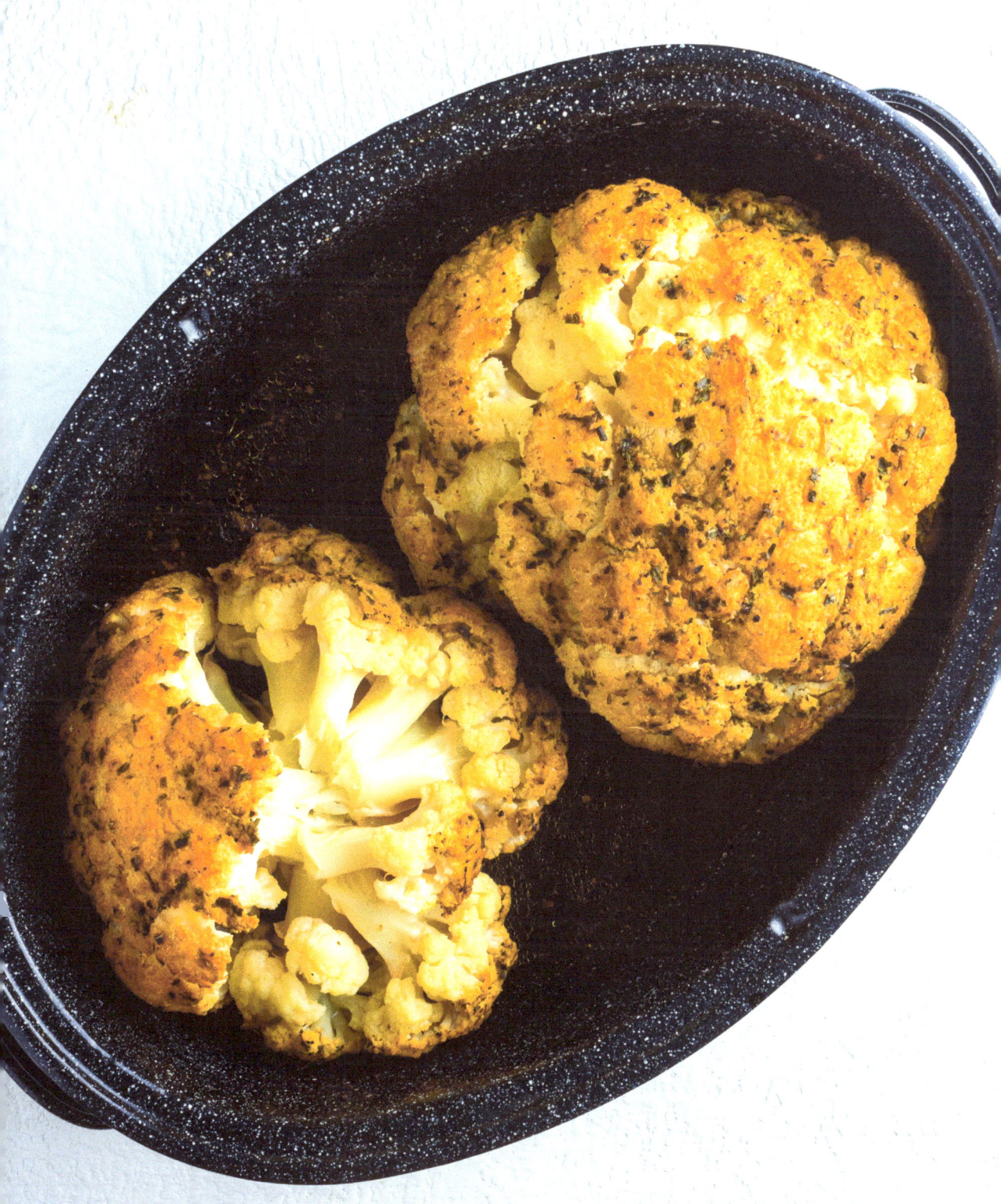

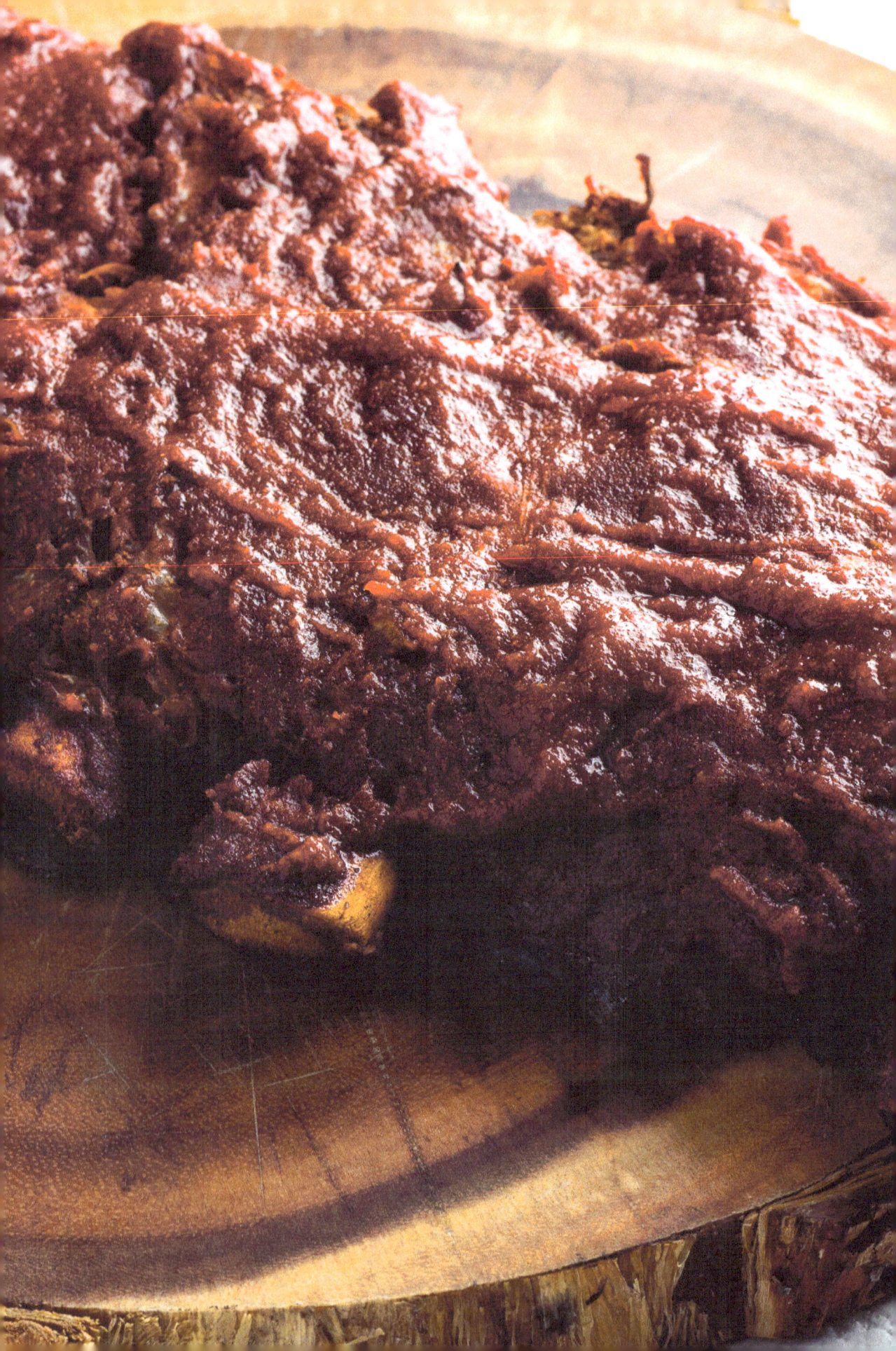

BARBECUE NIBS

INGREDIENTS

- 2 cans of Jackfruit
- 1 pack of King Oyster Mushrooms
- 4 cups walnut crumble or
- plant-based meat substitute
- 2 tbsp liquid smoke
- 2 tbsp liquid amino
- 4 tbsp paprika
- 2 tbsp smoked paprika
- 4 tbsp hamburger seasoning
- 2 tbsp seasoning salt
- 4 tbsp onion powder
- 2 tbsp. umami seasoning
- 6 tbsp. chia seeds
- 8 tbsp water
- 6 tbsp flax seeds
- 6 tbsp water
- 2 cups garbanzo flour
- 2 cups breadcrumbs
- 2 cups veggie broth
- 2 no beef bouillon cubes
- 2 cups breadcrumbs
- 1 cup barbecue sauce
- 1 Pack of thin Rice paper

INSTRUCTIONS

1. In a small bowl add flax seeds and six tbsp of water, set to side. In a separate bowl. Add chia seeds and eight tbsp of water, set to the side.
2. Open jackfruit, pour out brine, and transfer to a bowl of water. Remove any seeds. Soak for one hour then remove and drain in colander removing excess liquid. Pat dry with paper towel. Once complete dry lightly season with the dry spices above and let marinate.
3. Shred the end caps of oyster mushrooms with a fork then slice the tops.
4. In a medium pot bring two cups of veggie broth to a boil and add one no beef bouillon cube.
5. Add half of the seasonings and boil for two hours.
6. Remove from pot and transfer to a colander and let drain, removing all liquid.
7. In a medium bowl add jackfruit, walnut or meat substitute crumble, and shredded king oyster mushrooms. Mix well
8. A dd remaining dry ingredients and mix for 1-2 minutes, then add flax and chia.
9. Combine all ingredients thoroughly and add more seasoning as needed. Add more breadcrumbs if mixture does not stick together.
10. Dip rice paper sheets in a bowl of water and line them with the size of sheet tray. *Handle Gently*
11. Place mixture on the rice paper about ¼ thick. Cover the top of the mixture with the remaining rice paper.
12. Line a cookie sheet with parchment paper and create a ¼ inch thick rectangle. Place in freezer for at least five hours or overnight.
13. Remove from freeze. Grill each side for 3-5 minutes. (optional)
14. Remove from grill and transfer to cookie sheet lined with parchment paper.
15. Cover top of "ribs" with barbecue sauce.
16. Bake 15-20 minutes, then broil on low for 5-10 minutes or until crispy on top.

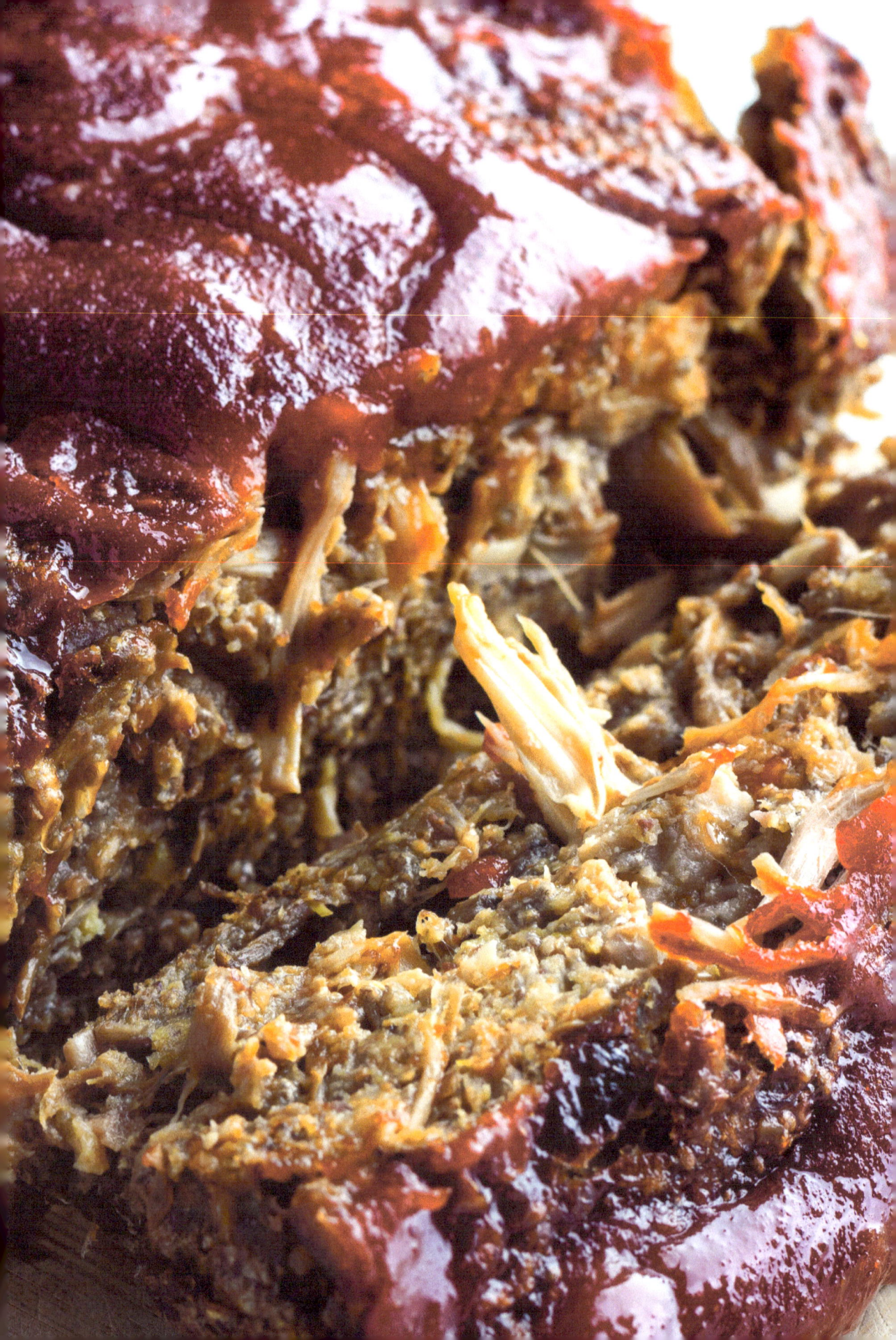

MEETLOAF

INGREDIENTS

- 1 pack of king oyster mushrooms
- ½ red bell pepper diced
- 2 tbsp seasoning salt
- 2 tbsp liquid smoke
- 4 tbsp paprika
- 4 tbsp hamburger seasoning
- 4 tbsp onion powder
- 6 tbsp. chia seeds
- 6 tbsp flax seeds
- 2 cups garbanzo flour
- 2 cups veggie broth
- 2 cups breadcrumbs
- 4 cups walnut crumble or plant-based meat substitute
- ½ yellow pepper
- ½ red onion diced
- ½ green pepper diced
- 2 tbsp. umami seasoning
- 2 tbsp liquid amino
- 2 tbsp smoked paprika
- 8 tbsp water
- 6 tbsp water
- 2 cups breadcrumbs
- 2 no beef bouillon cubes (optional)
- 1 cup barbecue sauce
- 1 Pack of thin rice paper
- 2 cans of Jackfruit

INSTRUCTIONS

1. Broil on low for 5-10 minutes.
2. Open jackfruit, pour out brine, and transfer to a bowl of water. Remove any seeds. Add Sea Salt and soak for at least two hours. Remove and drain in colander removing excess liquid. Pat dry with paper towel. Once complete dry lightly season with the dry spices above and let marinate.
3. Shred the end caps of oyster mushrooms with a fork then slice the tops.
4. In a medium pot bring two cups of veggie broth to a boil and add one no beef bouillon cube (optional).
5. Add half of the seasonings and boil for two hours or until tender.
6. Remove from pot and transfer to a colander and let drain, removing all liquid.
7. In a medium bowl add jackfruit, walnut crumble, or meat substitute crumble, and shredded king oyster mushrooms. Mix well, then add diced red onion, green, red, yellow, and green
8. Add remaining dry ingredients and mix for 1-2 minutes, then add flax and chia "egg".
9. Combine all ingredients thoroughly and add more seasoning as needed. Add more breadcrumbs if mixture does not stick together.
10. Line a loaf pan with parchment paper and transfer mixture.
11. Cover with foil and bake for 20-30 minutes then add barbeque sauce.

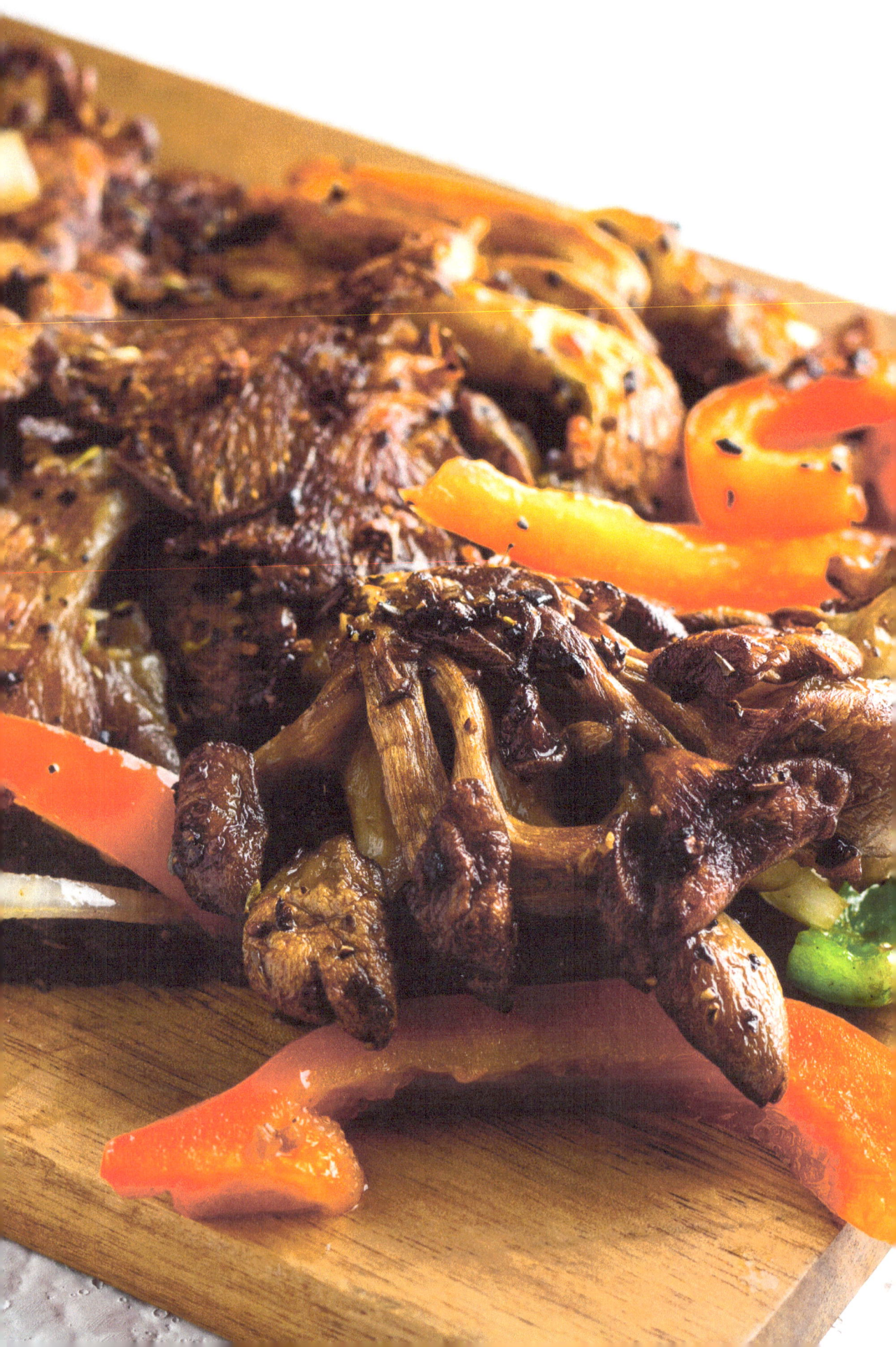

PAN SEARED OYSTER MUSHROOMS

If you knew me before I went plant-based, you'd know that steak was one of my favorite meats, and I loved how the fat on it burned just a little bit. I am sure some of you can relate! Ironically, this is in the group of things I let go first. Yes, I missed it and still do from time to time, which is what led me to create a plant-based version full of flavor. The texture of the king oyster mushroom is very "meaty" and the taste can mimic any of your favorites.

INGREDIENTS

- 2 Pack of Oyster Mushroom (big clusters work best)
- 1-2 Rosemary twigs
- 2 garlic cloves
- 2 tbsp plant-based butter
- 1 tbsp Worcestershire sauce
- 1 tbsp steak Seasoning
- 2 tbsp smoked paprika
- 1 tbsp Umami Seasoning
- ½ tsp ground black pepper
- 2 tbsp dried thyme
- 2 tbsp grapeseed oil

INSTRUCTIONS

1. In a cast iron skillet, heat grape seed oil on medium heat.
2. Add paprika, steak blend, and umami seasonings.
3. Add oyster mushrooms, then sprinkle with thyme, garlic cloves, and ground black pepper.
4. Place a heavy pot on another pan, preferably another cast iron skillet.
5. The heavier the pot, the easier to remove the moisture.
6. Cook for 3-5 minutes, then rotate.
7. Add butter and rosemary.
8. Cook for two to five minutes or until crispy on each side.

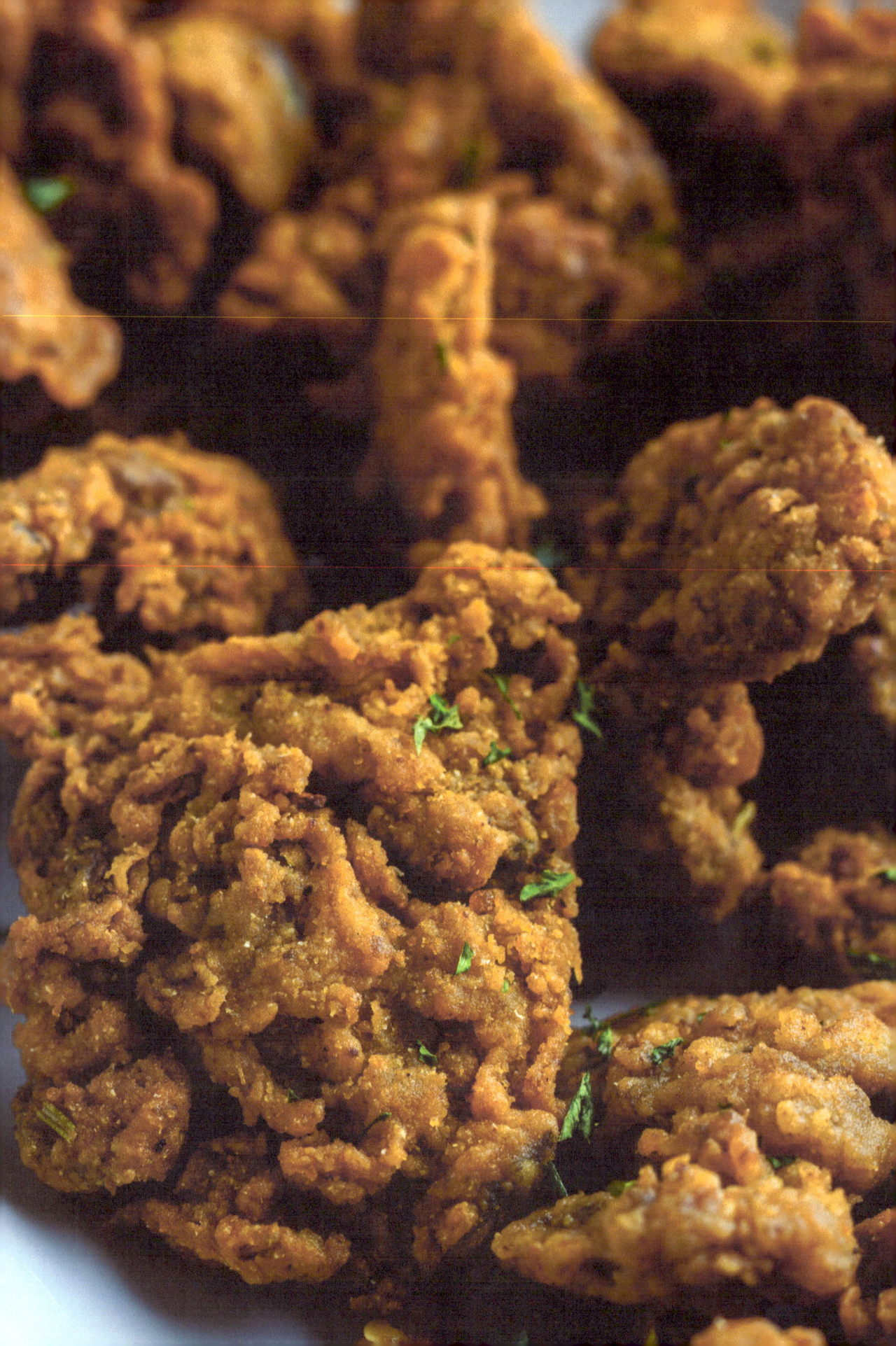

FRIED OYSTER MUSHROOMS

Trust me when I tell you anything you want to transform to plant-based is possible. If you are like me and love chicken, oyster mushrooms will be your go to for all things. I struggled for a very long time with chicken cravings. I love to be transparent so that it helps someone else on this journey. Season and fry them the same way you did before and pair then with your favorite sides.

INGREDIENTS

- 3-4 packs of oyster mushrooms
- 1 tbsp seasoning salt
- 4 cups of garbanzo flour
- 2 cups of plant-based milk
- 4 cups of unbleached all-purpose white flour (flour of choice)
- ¼ cup smoked paprika
- 2 tbsp paprika
- 1 tsp ground flax seed
- *Grapeseed Oil
- 2 tbsp chicken seasoning
- 2 tbsp black pepper

INSTRUCTIONS

1. Rinse mushrooms well and pat dry with a paper towel.
2. In a bowl add flax seeds and two tsp of plant-based milk and set aside.
3. In another bowl add garbanzo flour and in the last bowl add the unbleached white flour. Pour half of the dry ingredients into each bowl and mix to combine. Season flour well.
4. Dip mushrooms in wet batter, then unbleached flour(or flour of choice), then wet batter, then coat with garbanzo flour.
5. Turn deep fryer to 340° Fahrenheit and cook for 3-5 minutes or until crispy. Test temperature by sprinkling flour into grease. If it sizzles, the temperature is good.
6. Remove from grease and place on paper towel or cooling rack to drain grease.

*If you are using a deep fryer, please follow instructions for oil. If you are using a cast iron skillet, use one to two cups of grapeseed oil.

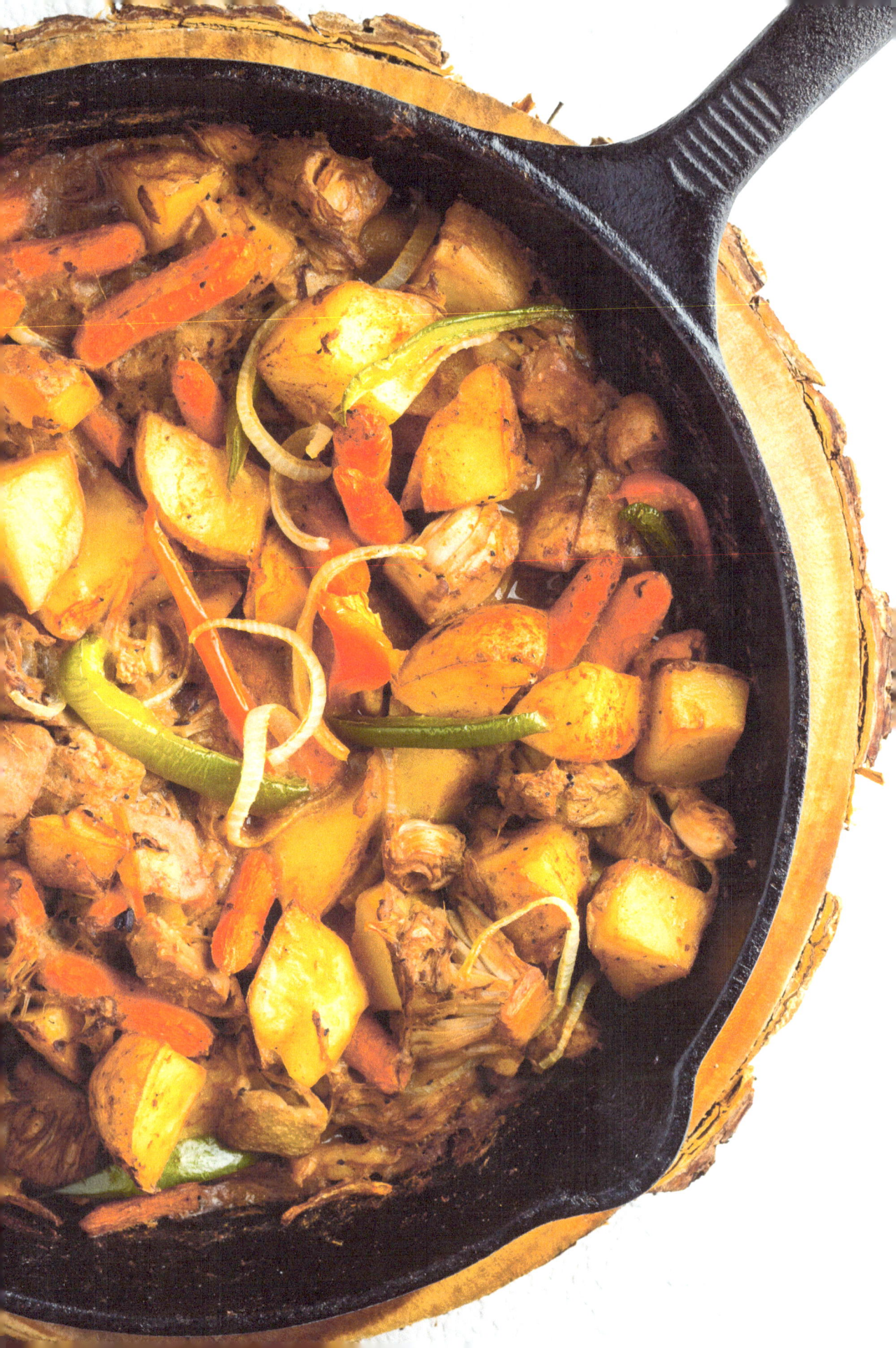

JACK FRUIT POTROAST

There's nothing like a good ole pot roast with some gravy, potatoes, and carrots. Hmmm, I can smell it now! This jackfruit pot roast does not disappoint. The entire family will enjoy this dish.

INGREDIENTS

- 2 cans of Jackfruit in brine
- ½ onion thinly sliced
- ½ tsp smoked paprika
- 1 tbsp steak seasoning
- ½ cup veggie broth or water
- 1 plant-based veggie bouillon cube
- 3-4 red potatoes
- ½ red bell pepper
- 1 tsp paprika
- 2 tbsp garbanzo flour
- ½ yellow pepper
- 1 bag of baby carrots
- ½ green pepper
- ½ tsp ground black pepper
- 2 tbsp grape seed oil
- ½ orange pepper

INSTRUCTIONS

1. Remove the jackfruit from the can and set aside. (Keep the pieces as whole as possible.
2. Soak in saltwater for at least six hours or overnight.
3. Pour into a colander and drain the water. Transfer to a bowl lined with paper towels and remove excess water.
4. Season jackfruit with liquid amino, liquid smoke, paprika, steak seasoning, and smoked paprika. Marinate overnight or at least six hours.
5. Preheat the oven to 350° Fahrenheit.
6. Rinse red potatoes, dry well. Dice into ¼ inch cubes.
7. Heat a cast-iron skillet on medium-high. Sprinkle a little steak seasoning to test the temperature. Once hot, add smoked paprika, black pepper, and paprika.
8. Add jackfruit and sear each side for 5–10 minutes before rotating. Sear the other side and add carrots. Cook for 15 minutes and add the red potatoes. Cook the potatoes for 5–10 minutes.
9. In a small bowl, whisk together the veggie broth and garbanzo flour until no lumps remain. Pour into a cast iron skillet. Taste and add more seasoning if needed. Cook until flour slushie thickens.
10. Add peppers to cast iron skillet then in the oven for 15-30 minutes or until potatoes and carrots are al dente.
11. Broil on low for 10-20 minutes or until top is browned and crispy.
12. Julienne the green, red, yellow, and orange peppers.
13. Add carrots, green, red, yellow, and orange peppers. Place the cast iron skillet in the oven and cook until the carrots are tender.
14. Remove from the oven and sprinkle with parsley(optional).

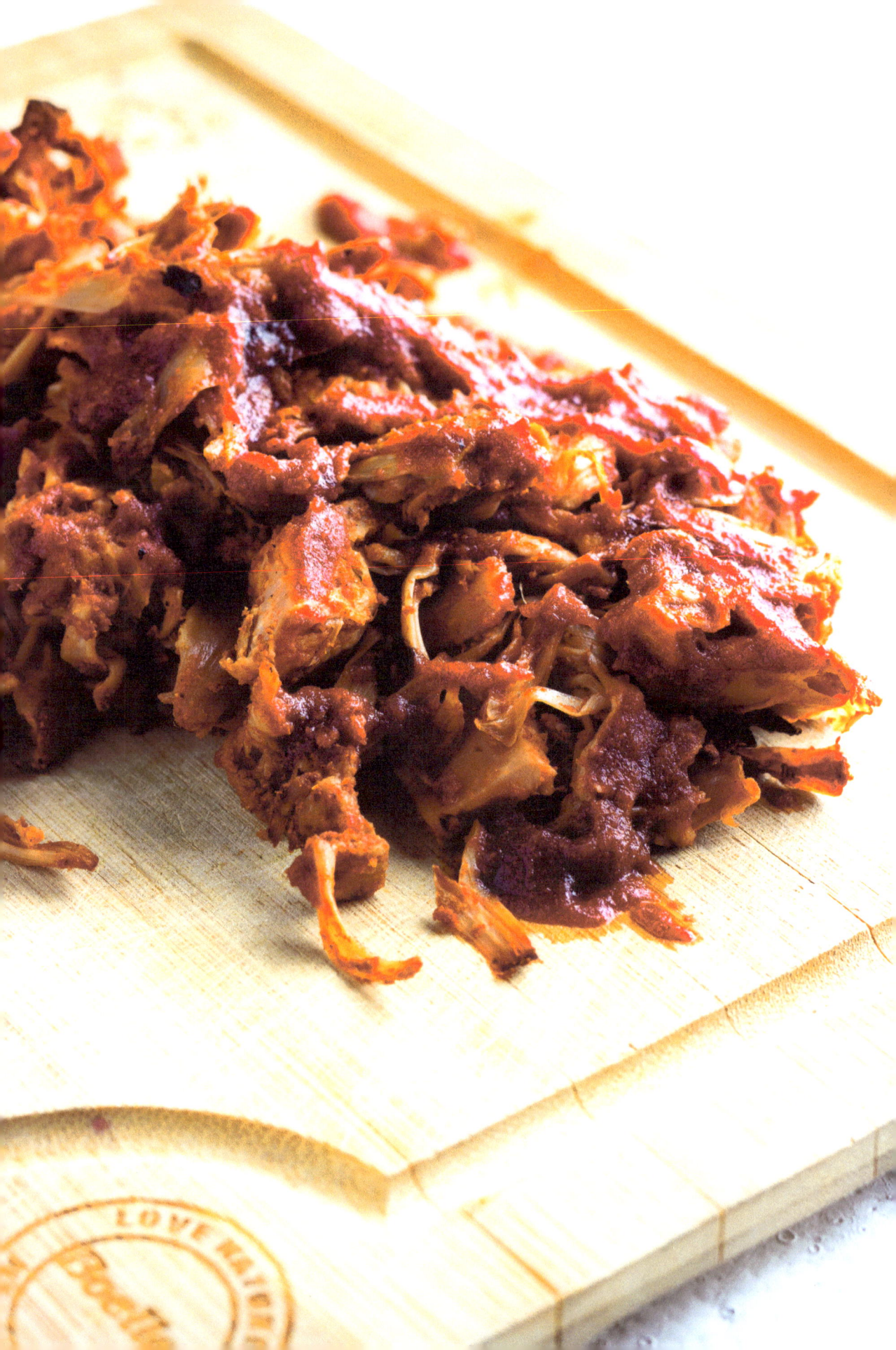

BARBECUE JACKFRUIT

INGREDIENTS

- 2 cans of Jackfruit
- 2 tbsp liquid smoke
- 2 tbsp paprika
- 2 tbsp seasoning salt
- 2 tbsp. umami seasoning
- 1 tbsp sea salt
- 2 tbsp liquid amino
- 4 tbsp smoked paprika
- 2 tbsp onion powder
- 1 cup of barbecue sauce

INSTRUCTIONS

1. Open the jackfruit and drain it in a colander, remove seed, then transfer to a bowl. Cover jackfruit with water, add sea salt. Soak for at least six hours or overnight.
2. Drain jackfruit in a colander, removing excess liquid. Pat dried with a paper towel. Lightly season with the dry spices and wet ingredients and marinate for at least six hours or overnight.
3. Remove from refrigerator. Check the jackfruit for seeds or hard parts and remove.
4. Preheat the oven to 425° Fahrenheit.
5. Line a cookie sheet with parchment paper. Spread the jackfruit evenly over the pan.
6. Bake for 25, then stir in the barbecue sauce. Bake for another 20-25 minutes, or until the jackfruit is crispy.

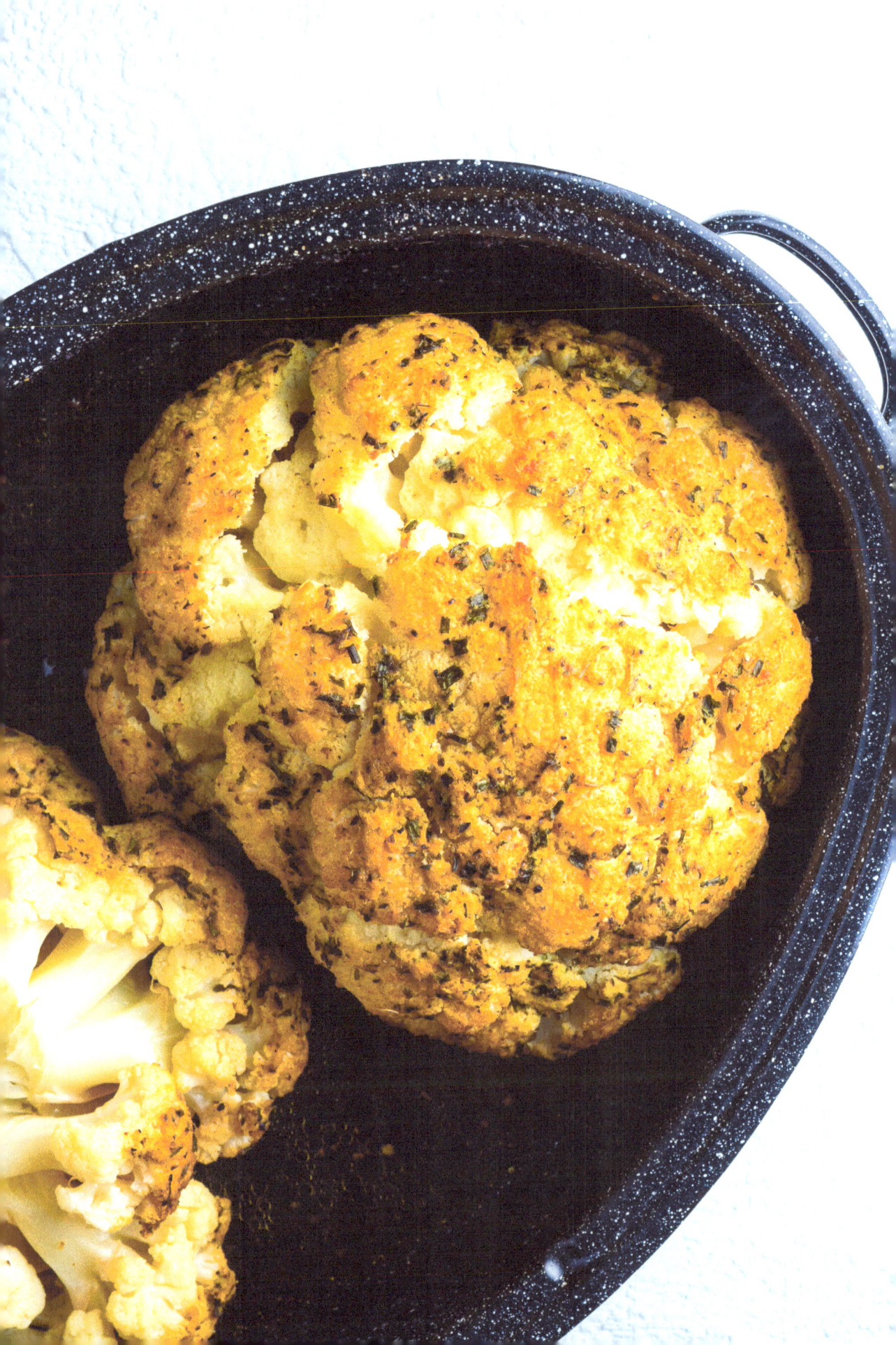

ROASTED CAULIFLOWER

INGREDIENTS

- 1-2 medium cauliflower
- 2 tbsp Dijon mustard
- 1 tbsp dried oregano
- 1 tsp onion powder
- ½ tsp ground black pepper
- ¼ cup grapeseed oil
- 2 tbsp white distilled vinegar
- 1 tsp dried chives
- 1 tsp salt, I use Sea salt
- ½ tps red pepper flakes

INSTRUCTIONS

1. Preheat the oven to 400º Fahrenheit.
2. Trim the outer leaves and cut the stem flush with the rest of the head so it can sit straight and then place the cauliflower in a deep roasting pan or Dutch oven.
3. Combine the rest of the ingredients in a glass measuring cup and mix well with a fork until well combined.
4. Pour that mixture over the cauliflower and rub it all over the cauliflower with your hands until it's completely coated.
5. Put the lid on and place it in the oven for 20–30 minutes, or until tender.
6. Take the lid off, set the oven to low broil, and cook for 5–10 minutes, or until golden brown.
7. Carefully transfer the fully cooked cauliflower to a plate and garnish with fresh chopped parsley and a drizzle of grapeseed oil.

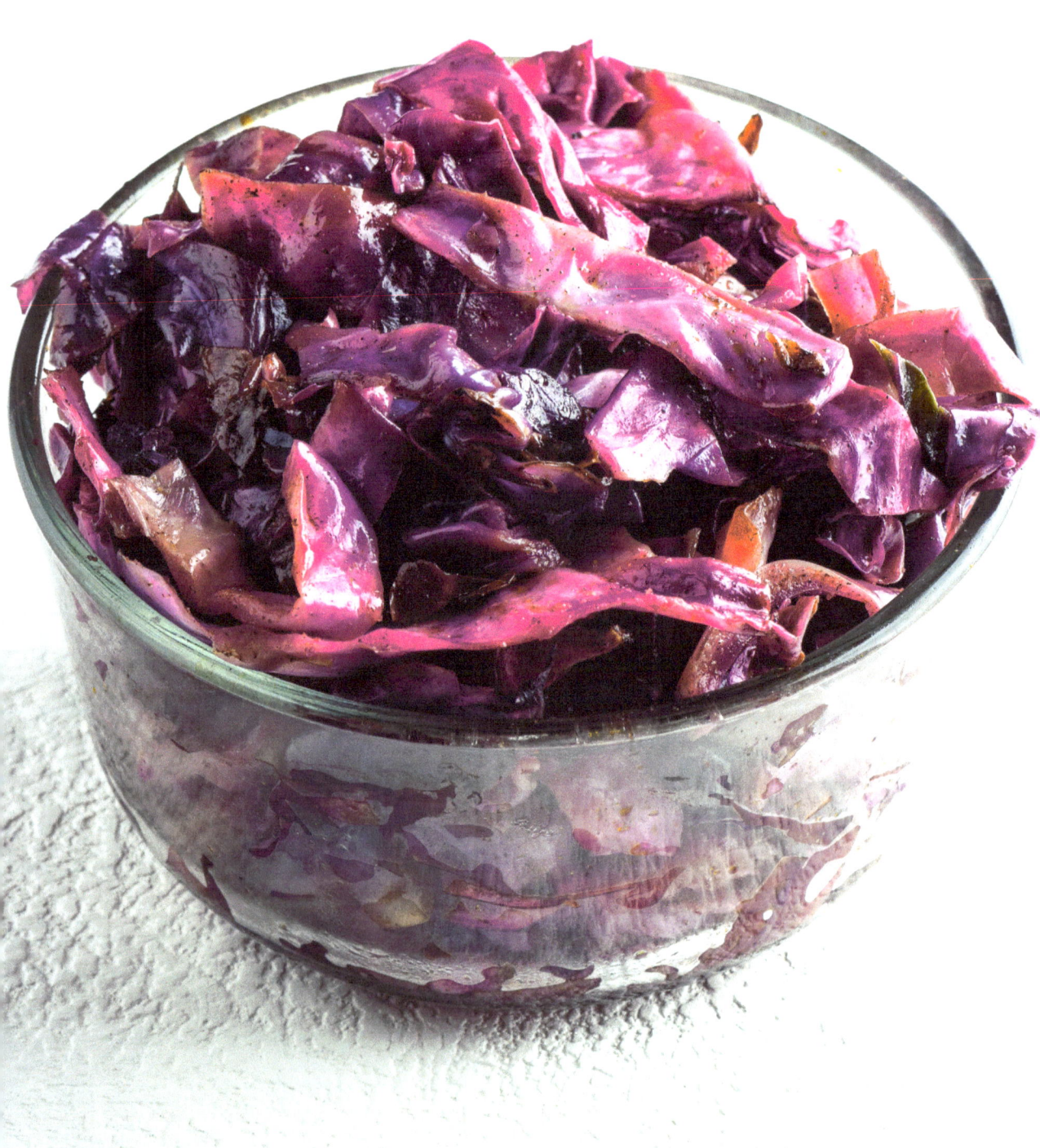

SIDE

DISHES

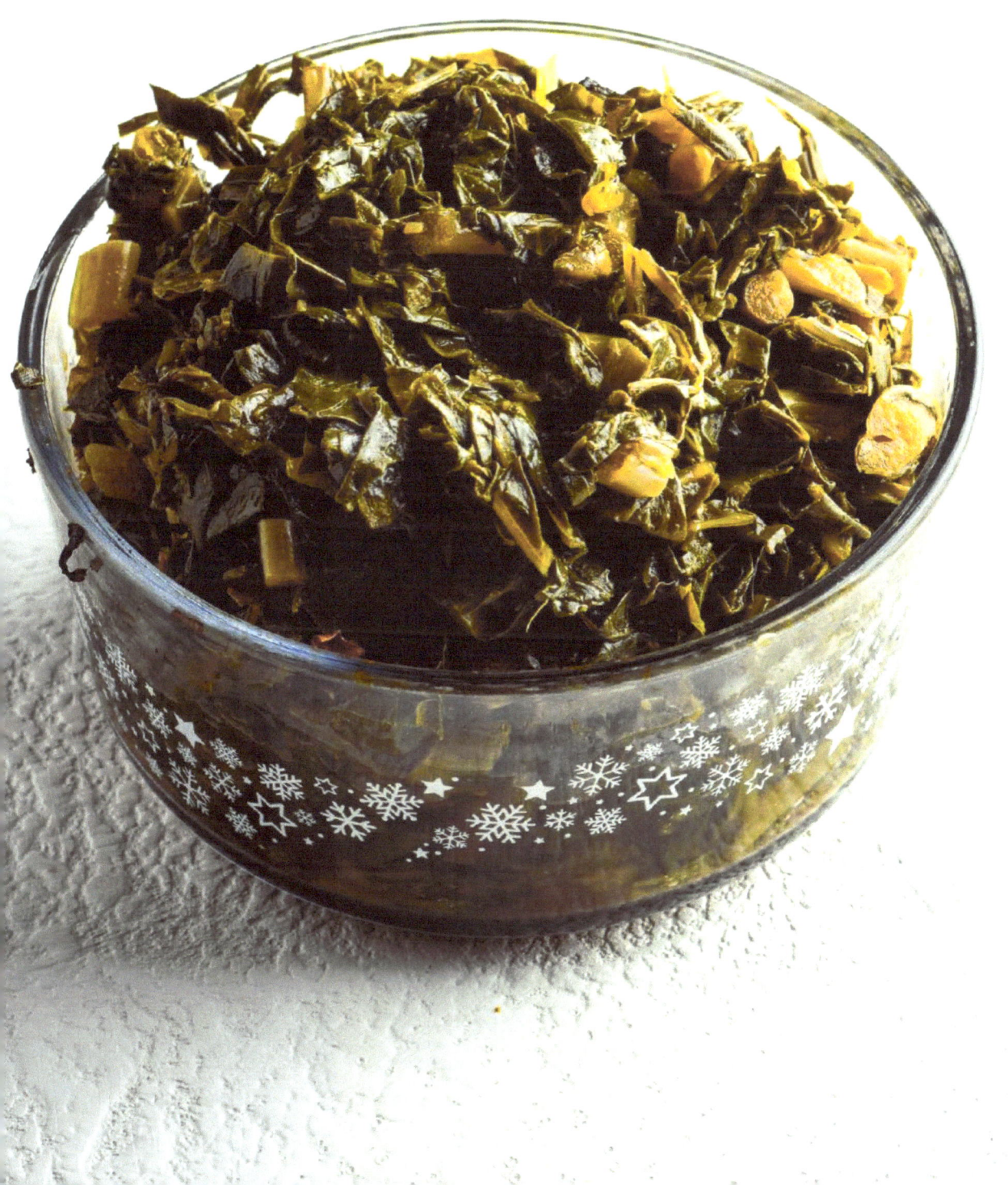

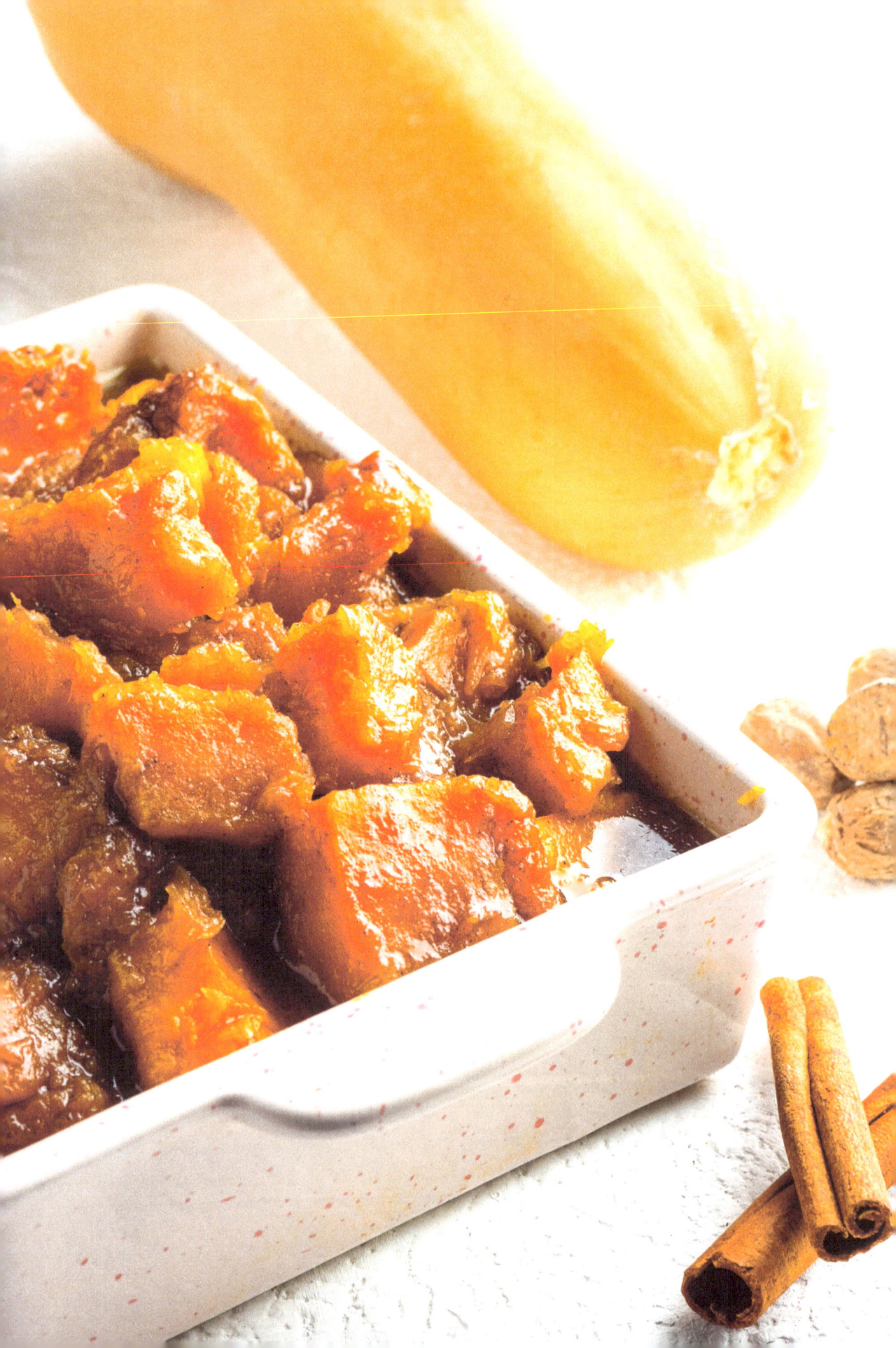

CANDIED BUTTERNUT SQUASH

If you are wondering, why squash allow me to introduce the benefits of this amazing vegetable. "Besides the usage of butternut squash for culinary, they have been abused for health benefits, which can be listed such as the ability to maintain the heart health, treat diabetes, boost the immune system, improve the bone and eye health, aid in weight loss, nourish hair and skin, etc."

INGREDIENTS

- 1 large Butternut Squash
- 1 tbsp cinnamon
- ½ cup brown sugar
- 1 tsp vanilla
- ⅛ tsp cardamom
- 1 tsp nutmeg
- 2 tbsp butter

INSTRUCTIONS

1. Pre-heat the oven to 400 Fahrenheit.
2. Place the squash in the oven for 20-30 minutes, or until a knife glides through. This helps cut the squash easily and decreases cooking time.
3. Remove it from the oven and set it aside to cool.
4. Once cooled, cut the top and bottom stem. Remove the skin and dice into ¼ inch cubes.
5. In a small skillet on low heat, add butter, cinnamon, brown sugar, cane sugar, vanilla, cardamom, and nutmeg. Stir until blended and smooth in consistency.
6. Add more sugar and spices according to taste.
7. Transfer to an 8x12 baking pan. Cover and place in oven.
8. Bake for 30-60 minutes, or until tender.

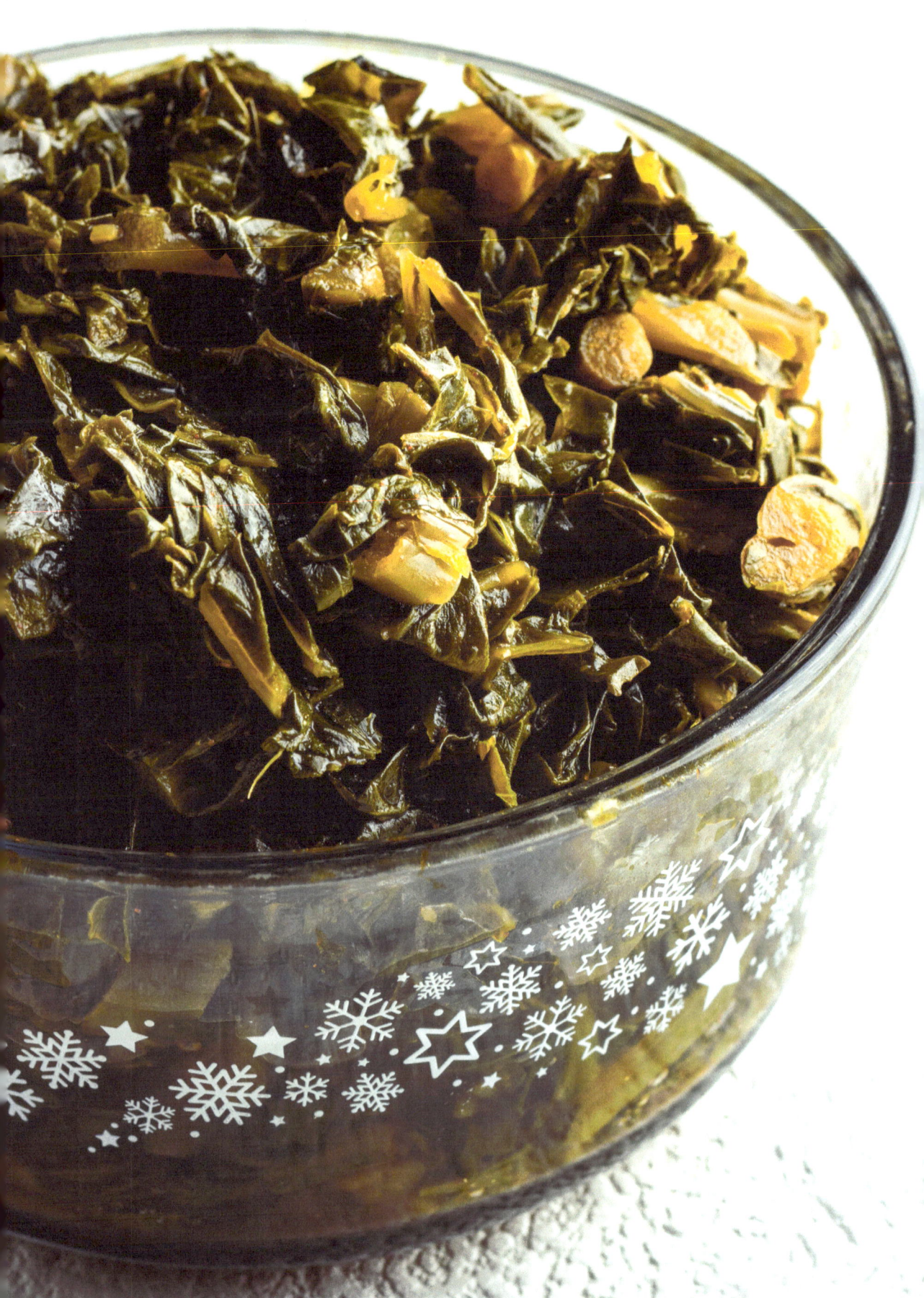

COLLARDS

INGREDIENTS

- 2 bags of shredded collard greens
- 2 tsp of liquid smoke
- 1 tsp garlic powder
- 1 tsp onion powder
- 2 tbsp liquid amino
- 1 tbsp Worcestershire sauce
- 2 tbsp smoked paprika
- 2 tbsp paprika
- 1 tbsp seasoning salt
- 4 cups vegetable broth
- 1 cup water
- 2 tbsp grapeseed oil

INSTRUCTIONS

1. Wash greens at least five times or soak for 45 minutes.
2. Pour the water and vegetable broth in the pot. When it comes to a boil add collard greens and seasoning.
3. Boil for two three hours or until tender.
4. Serve with sides. Add more seasoning if desired.

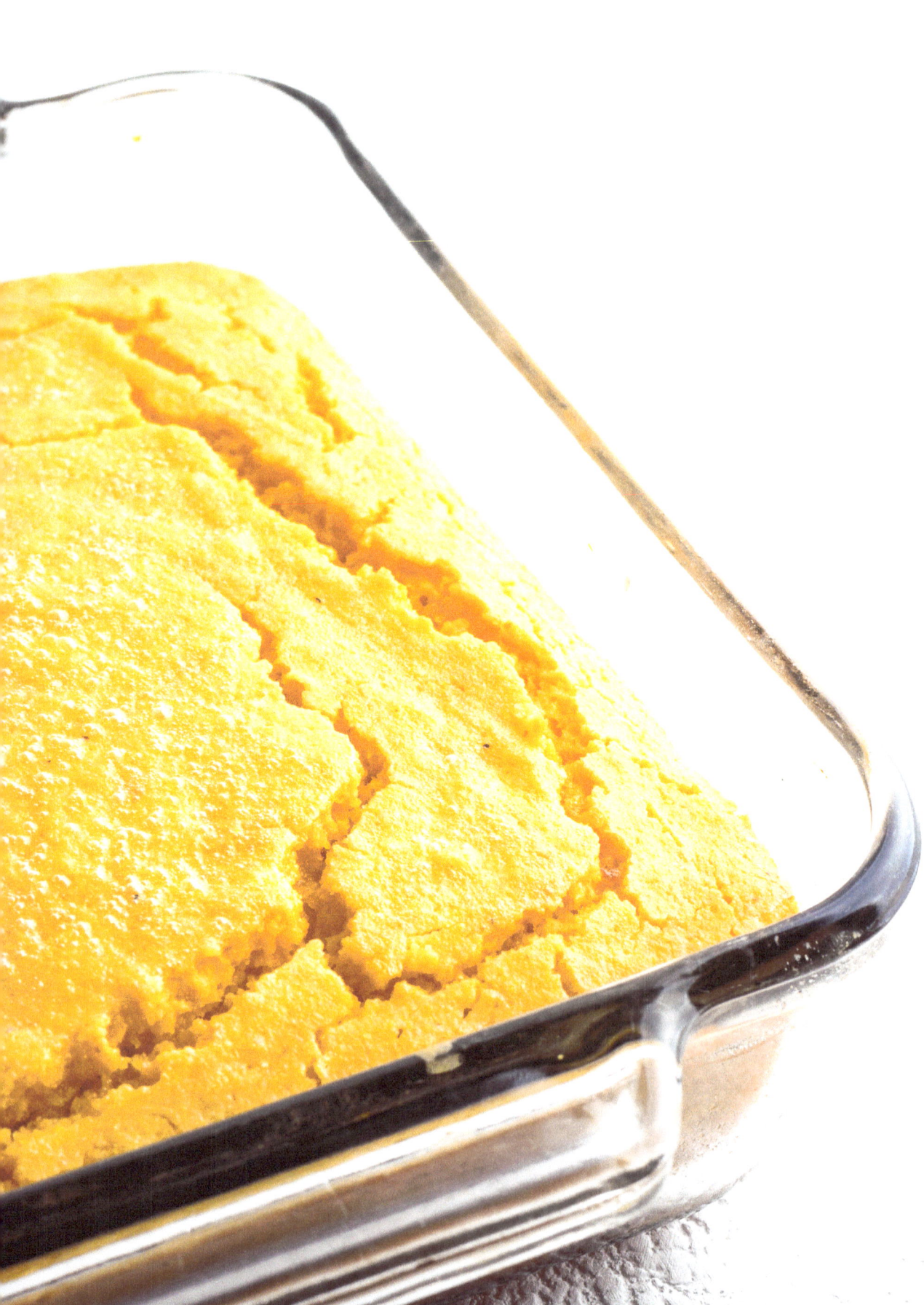

CORNBREAD

INGREDIENTS

- 1 ¼ cups plant-based milk
- ⅓ cup melted butter
- ½ cup maple or date syrup
- 1 cup cornmeal
- 1 ½ cups unbleached flour
- 1 tbsp baking powder
- 2 tbsp ground flaxseed
- 2 tbsp cinnamon
- ½ tbsp cardamom
- ½ tsp Celtic salt
- 4 tbsp room temperature butter
- 1/4 cup brown/date/coconut sugar

INSTRUCTIONS

1. Preheat oven to 400° Fahrenheit and lightly grease an 8x8 pan.
2. In a medium bowl, mix milk, syrup, coconut oil, and flaxseed.
3. Mix cornmeal, flour, baking powder, and salt in another bowl. Add milk mixture and stir until fully combined and the batter is smooth.
4. Pour the batter into the prepared pan, bake in the oven for 15-25 minutes or until a toothpick inserted in the center comes out clean.
5. Remove from oven, spread four tbsp room temperature butter on top (optional).
6. Let cool for 5-10 minutes then cut and serve.

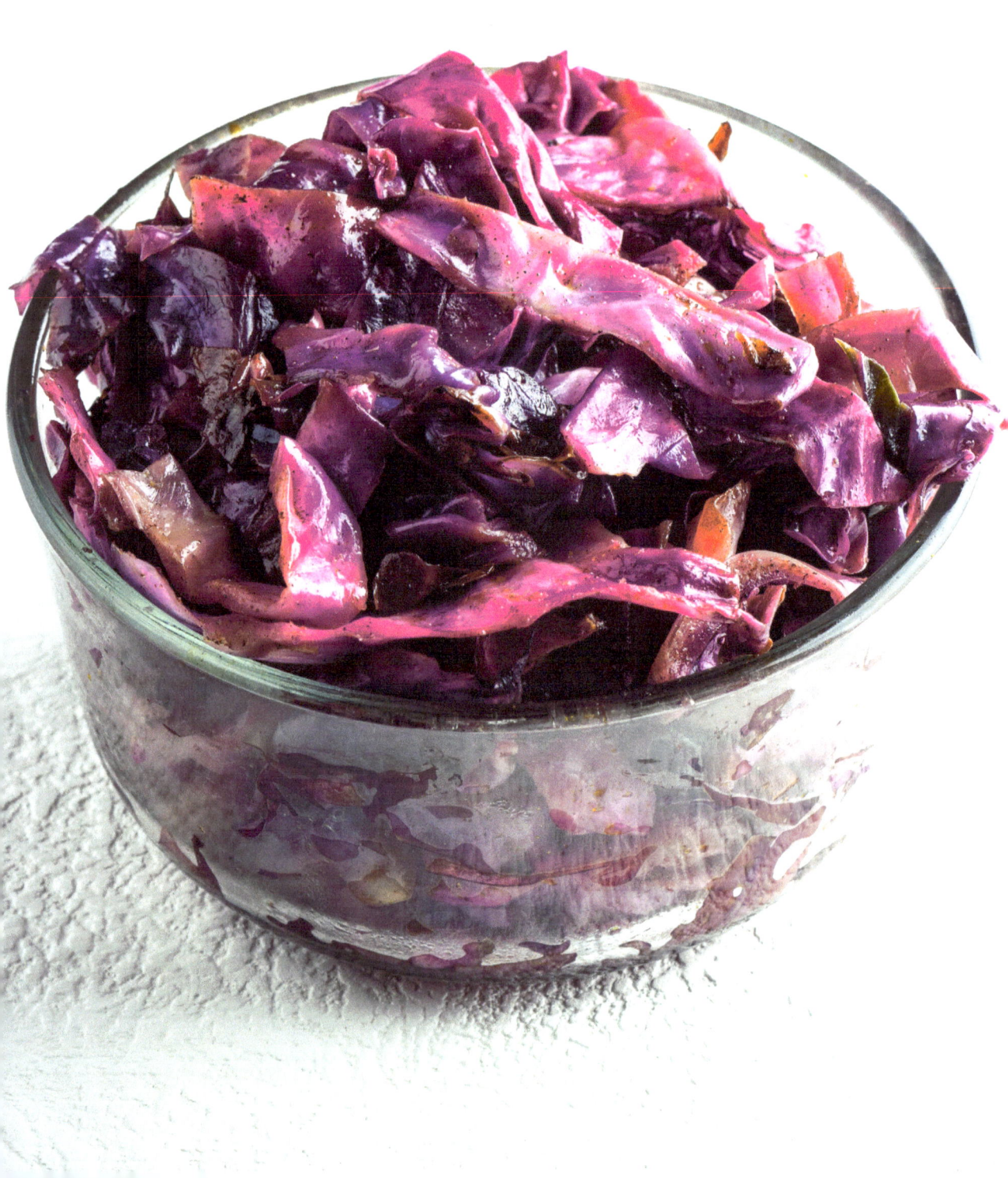

SAUTEED PURPLE CABBAGE

INGREDIENTS

- 1 large head of cabbage
- ½ cup vegetable broth
- 1 tbsp of smoked paprika
- 1 tbsp of onion powder
- 1 red onion
- 1 tbsp of paprika
- ½ tbsp of black pepper

INSTRUCTIONS

1. Remove any outside wilted leaves. Cut the end of the cabbage, then cut in half. Take one half and remove the bottom end including the white parts, repeat on the other half.
2. Julienne both halves of the cabbage.
3. Dice the red onion in ¼ inch cubes.
4. Sautee' onion in a cast iron skillet on medium high for about two minutes add water as need. This will create a broth. Add half of the herbs to the skillet and sauté cabbage for about 10-15 minutes or until tender.
5. Add more seasoning if desired.

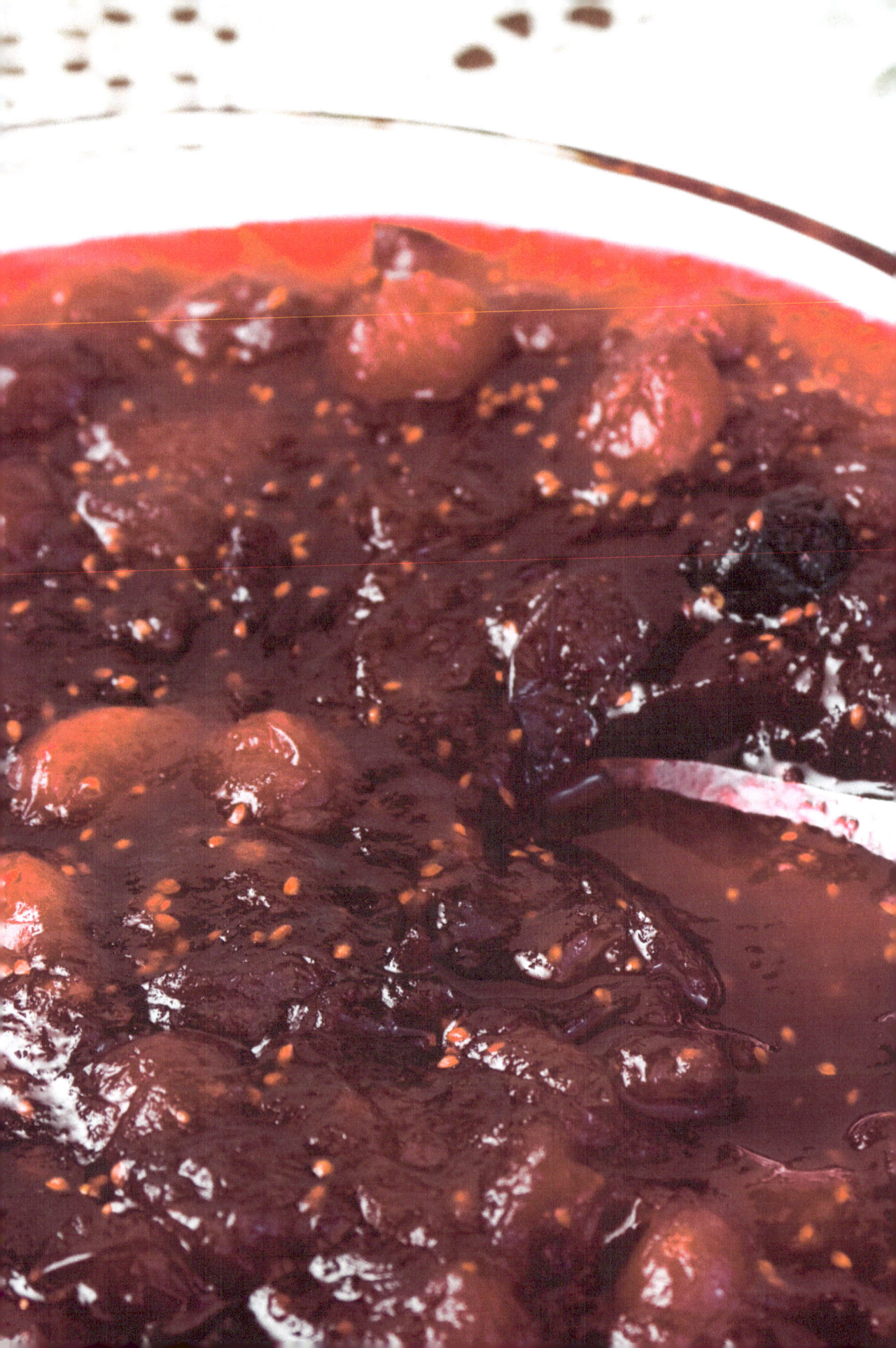

CRANBERRY SAUCE

INGREDIENTS

- 1 12oz package of fresh cranberries
- ½ cup date or maple syrup
- 1 tsp fresh squeezed mandarin juice

INSTRUCTIONS

1. Add the cranberries and syrup to a medium-sized saucepan and bring to a light boil over medium heat, stirring often. Pour in the mandarin juice.
2. Once the mixture comes to a boil, reduce the heat to low and continue cooking 10-12 minutes until the cranberries have burst and broken down and the thickened to your preference.
3. Remove from heat and let cool completely at room temperature. Chill in the fridge until ready to service.

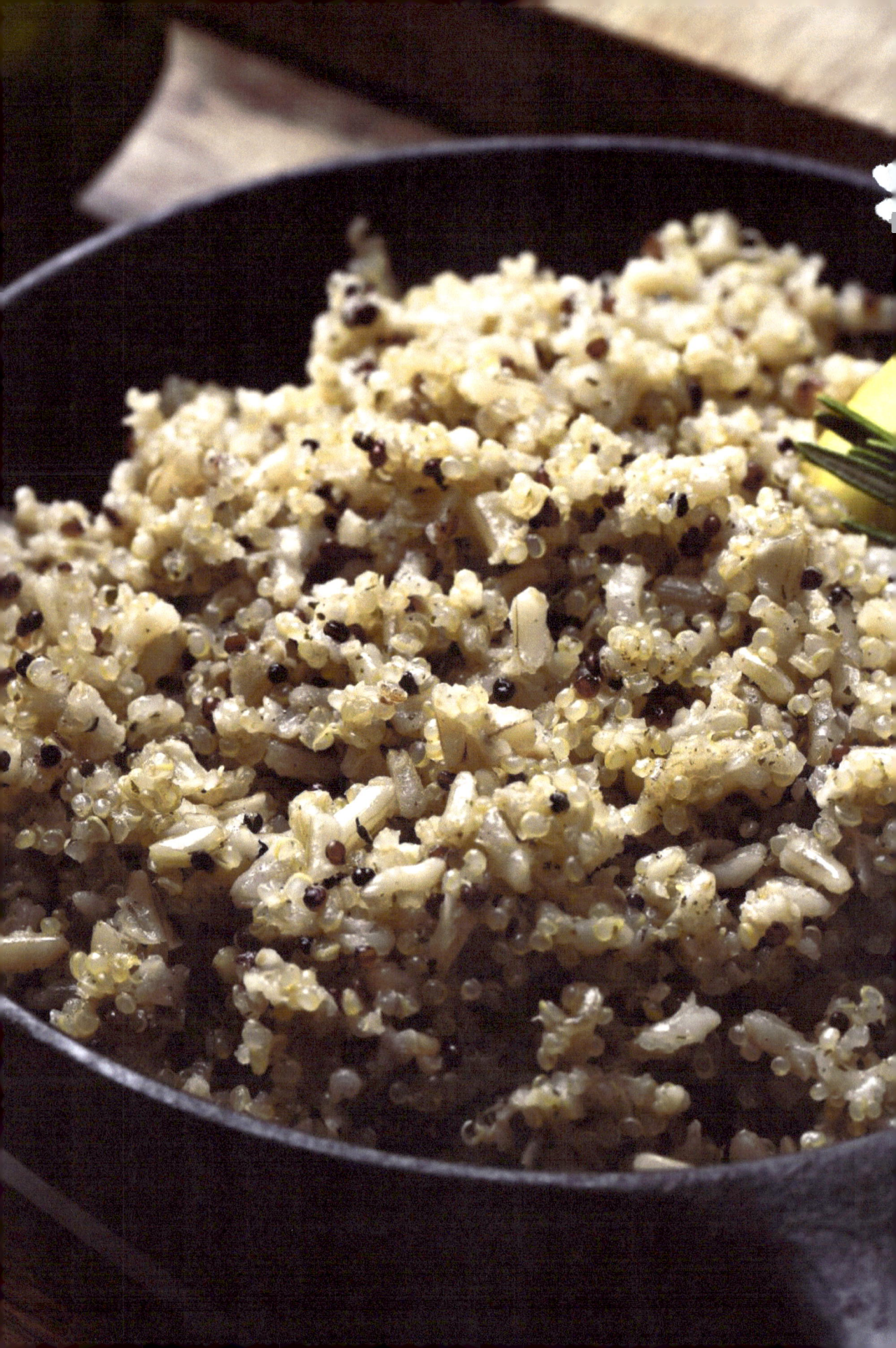

QUINOA

INGREDIENTS

- 2 cups quinoa
- 4 cups vegetable broth
- 1 tbsp onion powder
- Dash of sea salt
- 1 tbsp fresh cilantro

INSTRUCTIONS

1. In a medium pot heat vegetable broth on medium high. Bring to a boil and all ingredients. Cover and reduce to low and simmer for 15 minutes.
2. Remove lid, turn off heat, and fluff with a fork. Let cool for five minutes.
3. Garnish with fresh cilantro (optional).

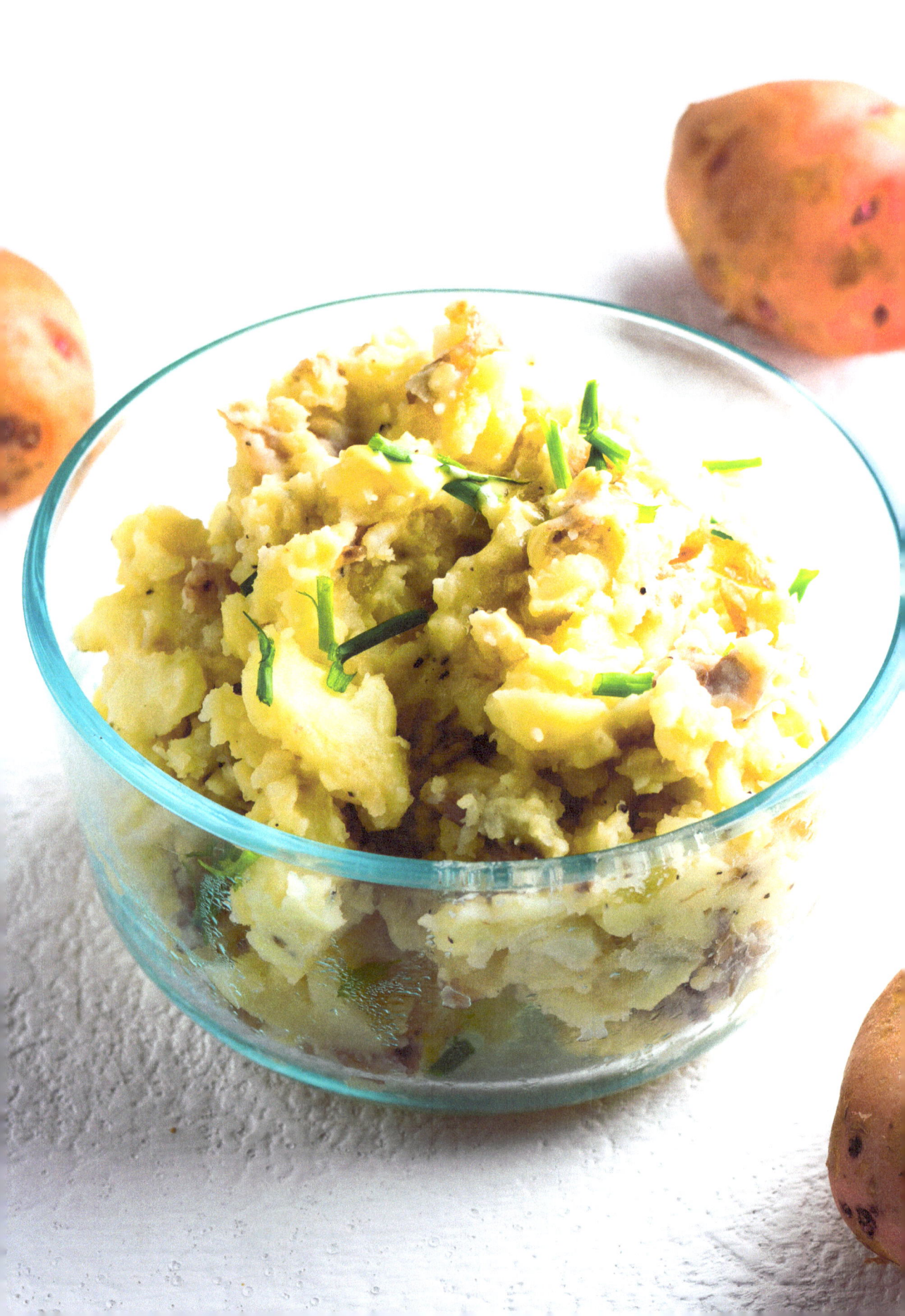

MASHED RED POTATOES

INGREDIENTS

- 4-8 Russet potatoes
- ½ cups plant-based milk
- 4 cups of water or potatoes are covered
- 4 tbsp of plant-based butter
- 2 garlic cloves
- ⅛ tsp salt
- ⅛ tsp pepper
- 1 tbsp fresh chives

INSTRUCTIONS

1. Wash potatoes and cut into medium diced pieces. Rinse diced potatoes and drain excess water.
2. In a medium to large pot add four cups of water. When water begins to boil add potatoes, butter, and garlic. Cook on medium high for 10-15 minutes or until tender.
3. Rinse potatoes with cold water and drain very well. Transfer to pot. On low heat add plant-based milk, salt and pepper. Add more butter if needed.
4. Stir all ingredients together until potatoes are mashed. Leave a few chunks.
5. Garnish with chives and serve.

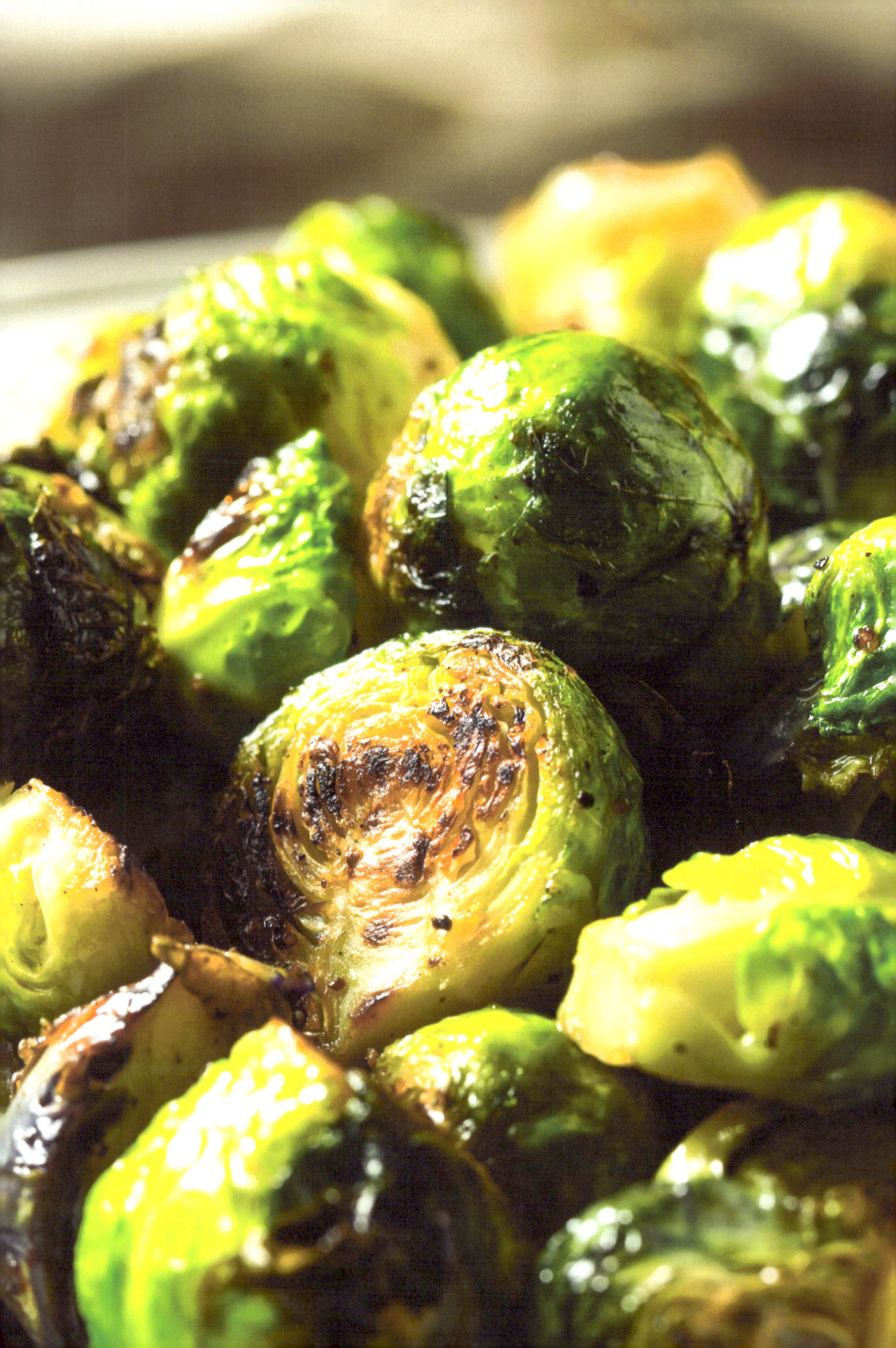

BALSAMIC GLAZED BRUSSEL SPROUTS

INGREDIENTS

- 1 12oz bag of whole Brussels sprouts
- 1 tsp ground black pepper
- 1 tbsp smoked paprika
- 1 tbsp balsamic vinegar
- ½ purple onion sliced
- ½ tbs season salt
- 1 tbsp paprika

INSTRUCTIONS

1. Preheat the oven to 425° Fahrenheit.
2. Wash and pat dry Brussels sprouts dry.
3. Cut bottom of brussels sprouts then cut in half and place them on a baking sheet pan lined with parchment paper. Massage all the spices into the Brussels.
4. Dice purple onion into medium sized dices.
5. Cook for 10 minutes, then rotate and cook for another 10-15 minutes, or until crispy.
6. Transfer to a plate and drizzle with balsamic glaze and balsamic vinegar.

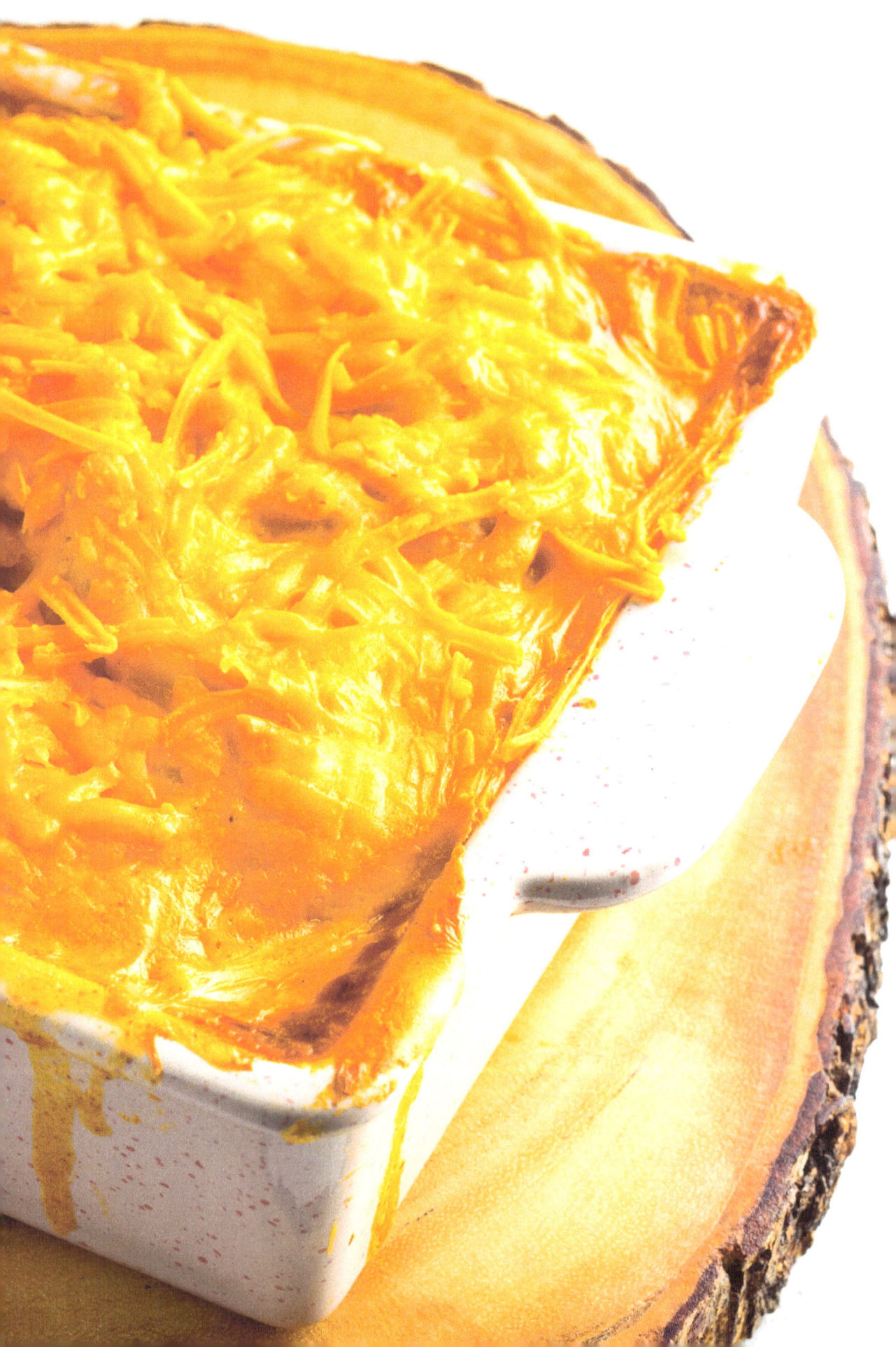

MAC 'N CHEEZE

It took me five years to master macaroni and cheese. I made it every possible way before realizing I was doing too much and decided to go back to the basics of when I made non-plant-based macaroni. I got in the kitchen one day, got a groove going, took a deep breath, consulted with the ancestors and made magic. I am so in love with this Mac and cheese and there is no doubt you and your family will enjoy it.

INGREDIENTS

- 1 16 oz box of elbow noodle
- 2 16 oz bag of shredded cheddar cheeze
- 4 slices of American cheeze (not cheese)
- 2 cups pasta water
- 2 tbsp paprika
- 1 tbsp ground black pepper
- 2 tbsp c smoked paprika
- ¼ cup nutritional yeast
- 2 16 oz bag of shredded mozzarella cheeze
- 4 tbsp sour cream
- 1 cup plant-based milk
- ½ tsp yellow mustard
- ½ tbsp onion powder
- 2 cups of water

INSTRUCTIONS

1. Add the water to a large-sized saucepan and bring to a light boil over medium heat. Pour in the elbow noodles. Cook for six minutes, rinse with cold water to slow cooking.
2. Place a bowl under the colander to preserve the pasta water. Pour two cups in the pot. Add one bag of cheddar/mozzarella cheeze and the sliced cheeze.
3. Cook for 30 minutes or until cheese sauce thickens. Add milk and stir well.
4. Preheat oven to 400° Fahrenheit.
5. Add onion powder, nutritional yeast, paprika, smoked, paprika, and seasoning salt.
6. Mix well, taste and add more seasoning as needed.
7. In a large baking pan add noodles, sour cream, and black pepper. Stir well.
8. Pour cheese blend into pan and mix well. Cover with the remaining shredded cheeze.
9. Cover with foil and back for 10-15. Remove foil and broil on low for 5-10 minutes or until cheeze is melted and brown.

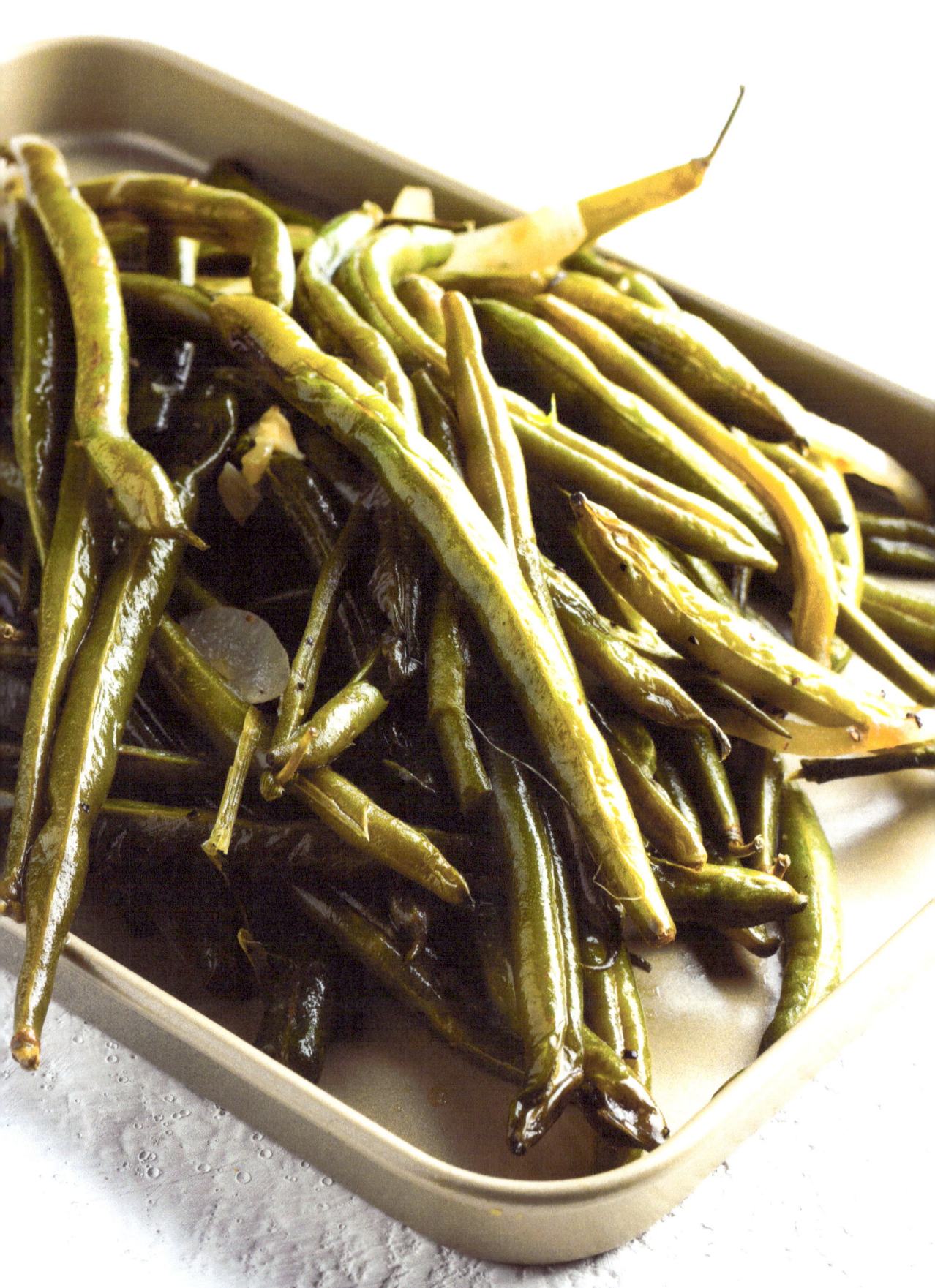

GREEN BEANS

INGREDIENTS

- 1 bag of green beans
- 2 garlic gloves
- ½ white onion
- 1 tsp black pepper
- ½ tsp liquid smoke
- ½ tsp liquid amino
- ½ tsp smoked paprika
- ¼ cup vegetable broth

INSTRUCTIONS

1. Wash green beans in colander and let dry.
2. Thinly slice half of white onion.
3. Flatten garlic with knife (this releases more flavor), then dice into fine pieces and set aside.
4. Heat cast iron skillet on medium high.
5. Add green beans, onion, and garlic. Sautee for 5-10 minutes then add vegetable broth.
6. Cook for 5-10 minutes. I prefer al dente.

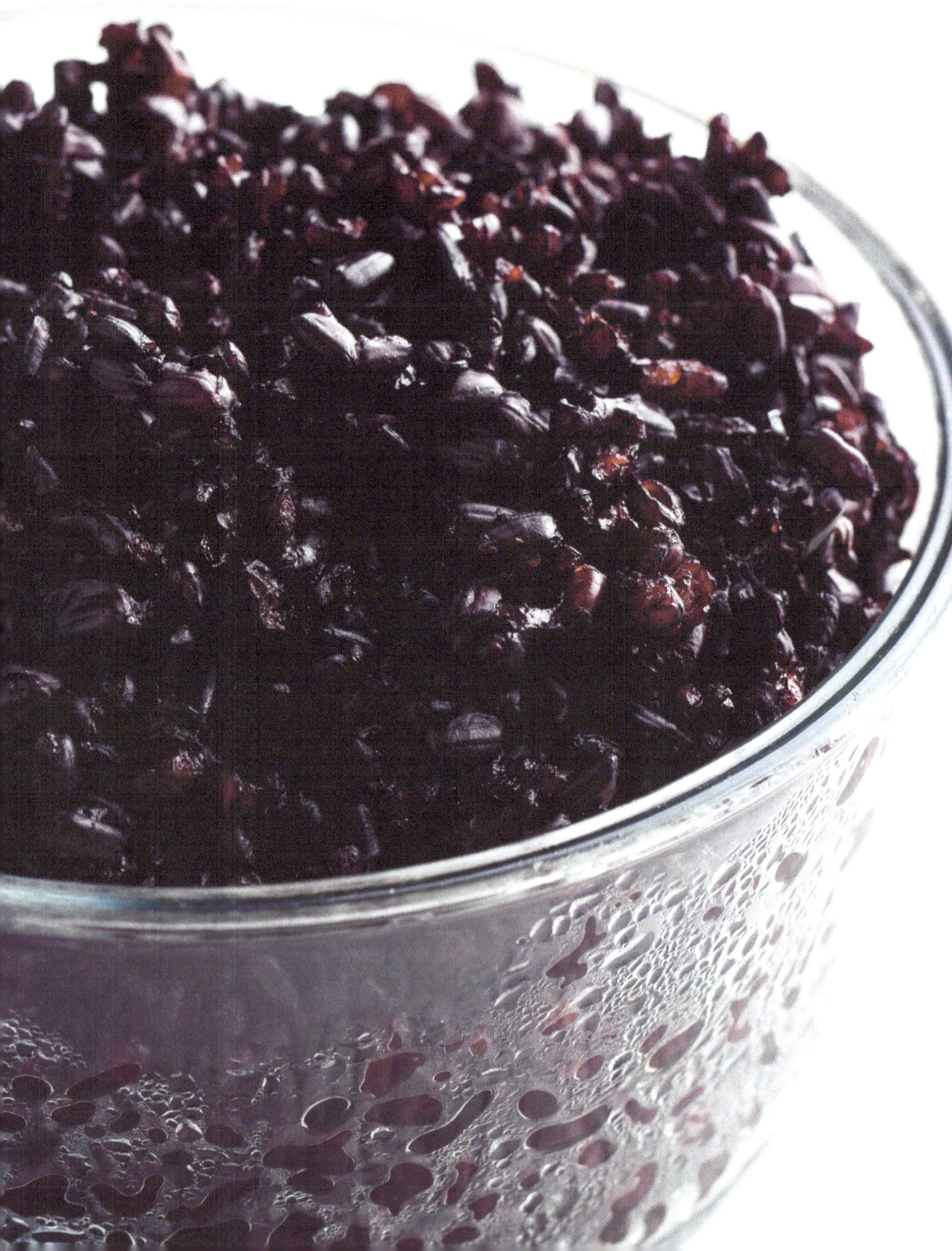

BLACK RICE

Also known as forbidden or purple rice, black rice is a type of rice that belongs to Orzo sativa. In ancient China, it's said that black rice was considered so unique and nutritious that it was forbidden to all but royalty. Compared with other types of rice, black rice is one of the highest in protein. In addition to being a good source of protein, fiber, and iron, black rice is especially high in several antioxidants. Anthocyanins from black rice may also have potent anticancer properties. A review of population-based studies found that higher intake of Anthocyanins-rich foods was associated with a lower risk of colorectal cancer. Black rice contains high amounts of lute in and zeaxanthin, two types of arytenoids that are associated with eye health. " 2019 (K.McGrane RS, RD).

INGREDIENTS

- 1 cup black rice
- 2 cups veggie broth

INSTRUCTIONS

1. Soak rice for 45 minutes to an hour (this helps it cook quicker).
2. Heat pot on medium high and add veggie broth. When broth boils add rice and cover.
3. Cook for 30 minutes, remove lid and check texture. If rice needs more time, cover and cook for 10-15 minutes or until tender.

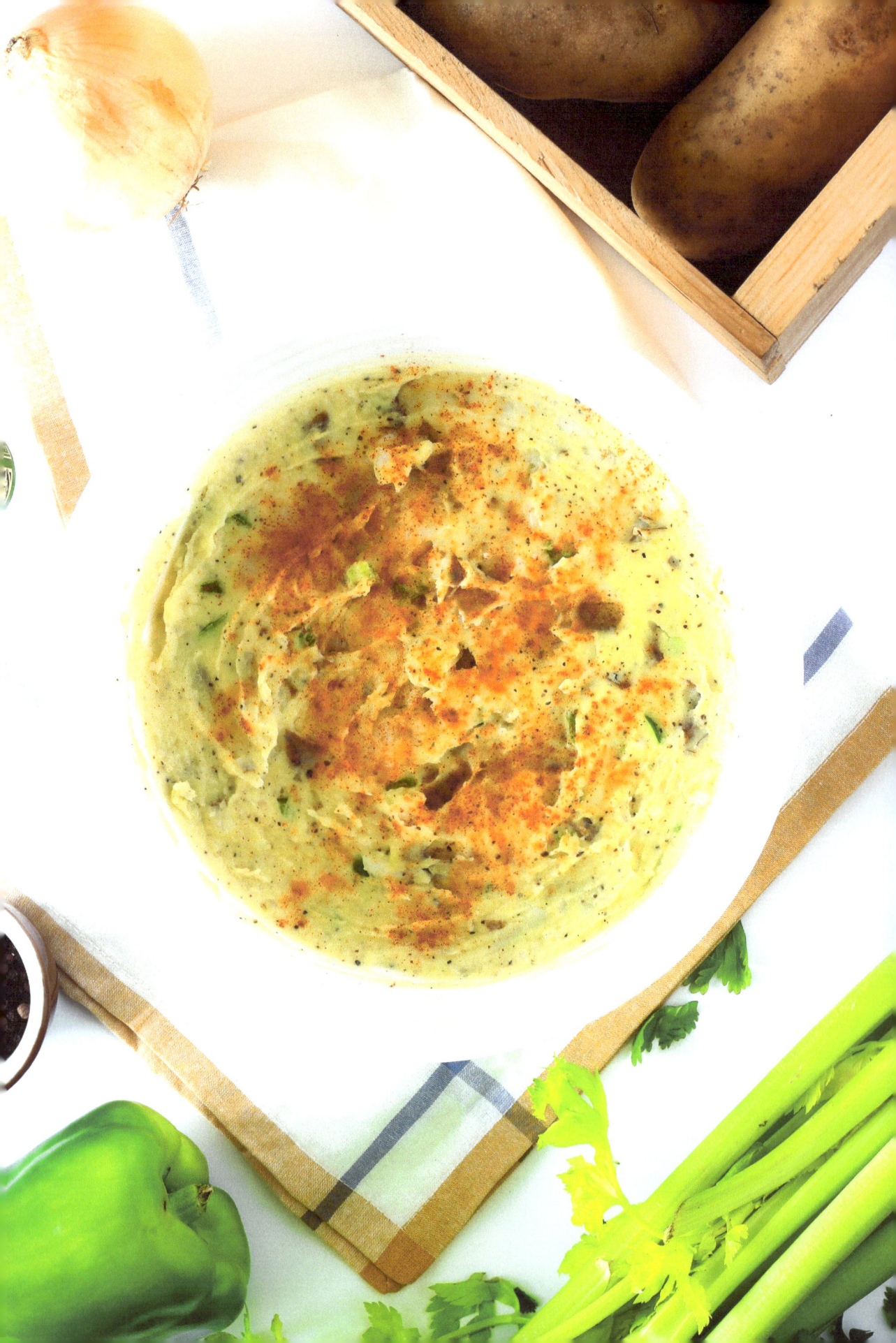

POTATO SALAD

This recipe is in the first cookbook, "35 Days, 35 Ways Delicious Recipes for the Vegan Lifestyle," but I decided to include it because.
1. What is a menu without potato salad and
2. I have elevated the recipe and wanted to share.

The only potato salad I have ever loved is my moms' and mine. The last recipe was missing one key ingredient and now that I found it, this recipe is 100% close to my moms'. The secret is black salt, it has an egg like smell and taste. I can't wait for you to taste it.

INGREDIENTS

- 4 Russet potatoes
- 1 tbsp diced celery or celery seeds
- 4 tbsp green pepper
- ½ cup plant-based mayo
- ⅛ tsp black pepper
- ¼ tsp black salt
- 4 cups of water or until potatoes are covered
- 4 tbsp onion
- 2 tbsp yellow mustard
- Dash of sea salt
- Dash of paprika

INSTRUCTIONS

1. Wash potatoes and cut into medium diced pieces. Rinse diced potatoes and drain excess water.
2. In a medium to large pot add four cups of water. When water begins to boil add potatoes. Cook on medium high for 10-15 minutes or until tender.
3. Rinse potatoes with cold water and drain very well. Transfer to mixing bowl.
4. Add potatoes, mayo, mustard, chopped celery or celery seeds, diced onion, sea salt, pepper, paprika, green pepper, and black salt.
5. Stir all ingredients together until you have a nice light-yellow color. You may need to add more mustard according to taste and color.
6. Cover with plastic wrap and place in fridge for one to two hours. Serve cold or warm.
7. Garnish with smoked paprika (optional).

DESS

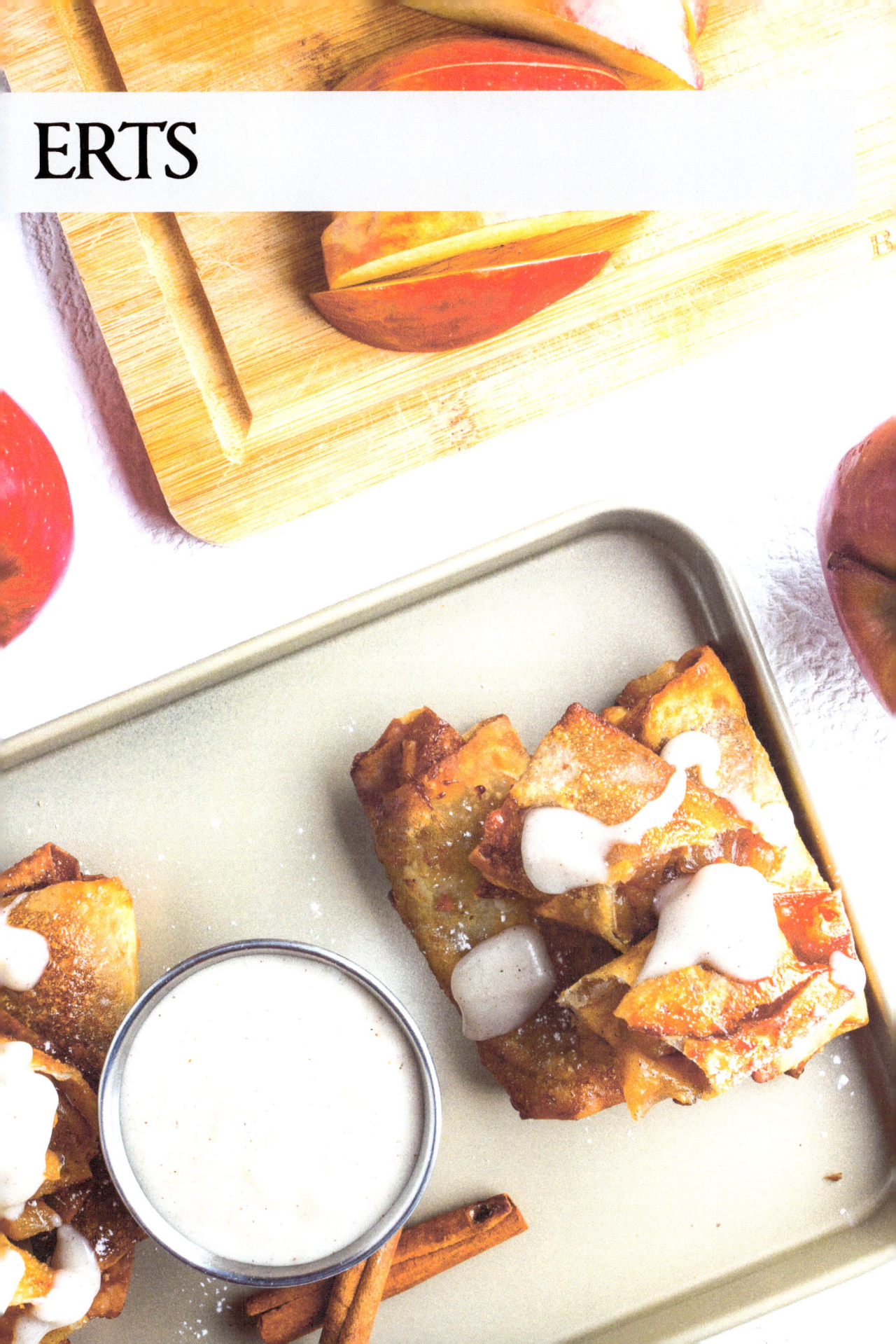

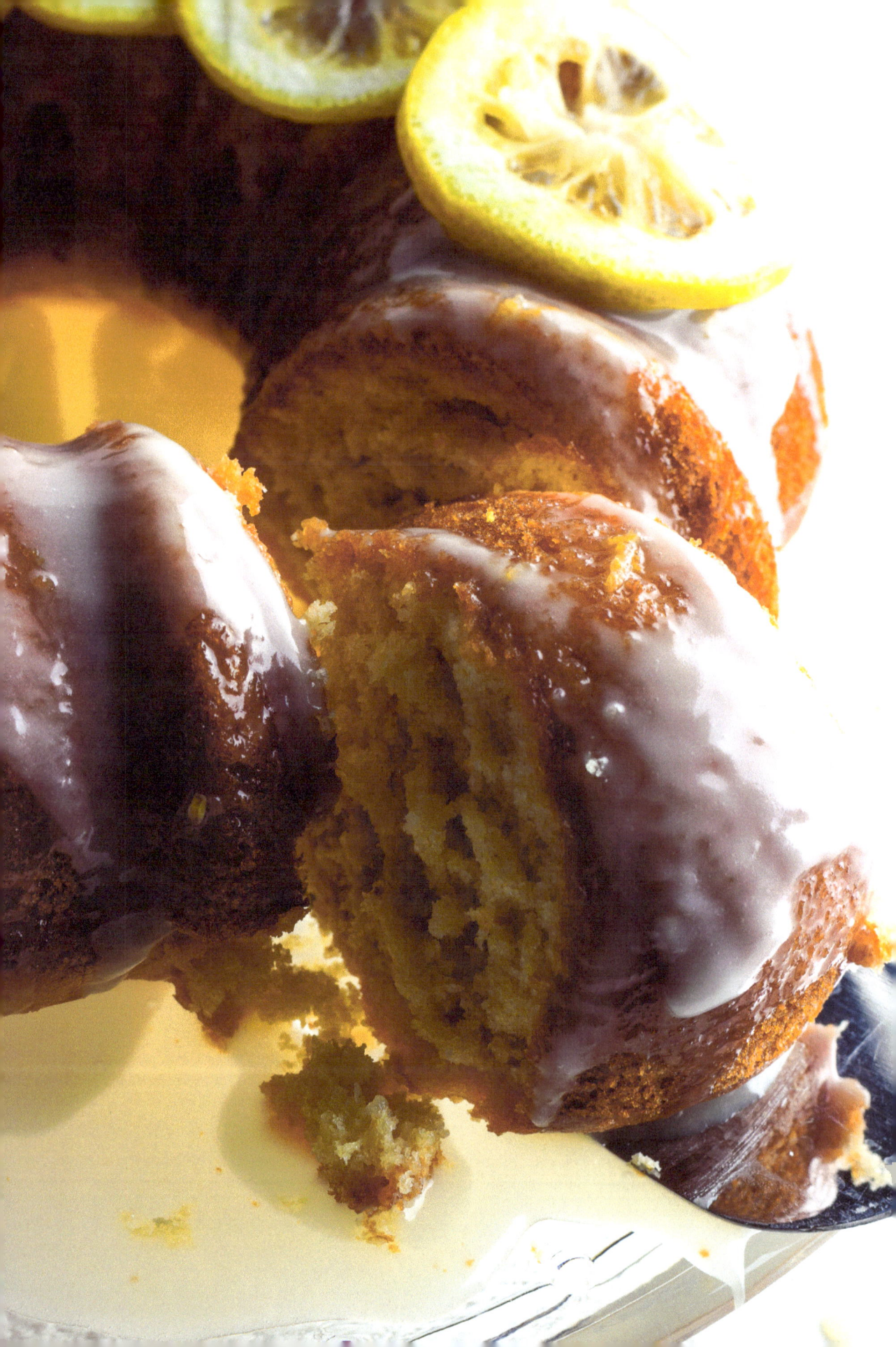

LEMON BUNDT CAKE

This recipe is also in my previous cookbook "35 Days, 35 Ways Delicious Recipes for the Vegan Lifestyle." I added it because this recipe is elevated and is a favorite anytime of the year. Why not add it to the plant-based spread. I love a good ole lemon cake with some ice cream aka nice cream!

INGREDIENTS

- 1 cup milk of choice (I used Not Milk)
- ½ cup fresh squeezed lemon juice
- 1 tsp vanilla extract
- 1 tsp lemon zest
- 1 cup cane sugar
- ¼ cup melted butter
- 1 ½ tsp baking powder
- 2 ¼ cup unbleached all-purpose flour

Lemon Frosting

- 1 ½ cups powdered sugar
- ¼ cup softened butter
- ¼ cup cream cheese
- 1 tsp cinnamon
- 1 tsp cardamom
- 2-4 tbsp fresh lemon juice

INSTRUCTIONS

1. Preheat oven to 375⁰ Fahrenheit.
2. Mix (by hand) the lemon juice, melted vegan butter, vanilla, milk, sugar. Add 1 tsp of lemon zest for a bolder lemon flavor. Add baking soda and baking powder and mix. The mixture will bubble. Next add the flour and mix until smooth.
3. Pour the batter into a greased Bundt back and bake for 20-25 minutes or until golden brown with a crisp top.
4. While the lemon cake is backing, use a whisk to mix the cream cheese icing ingredients and spread over the warm or cooled cake.

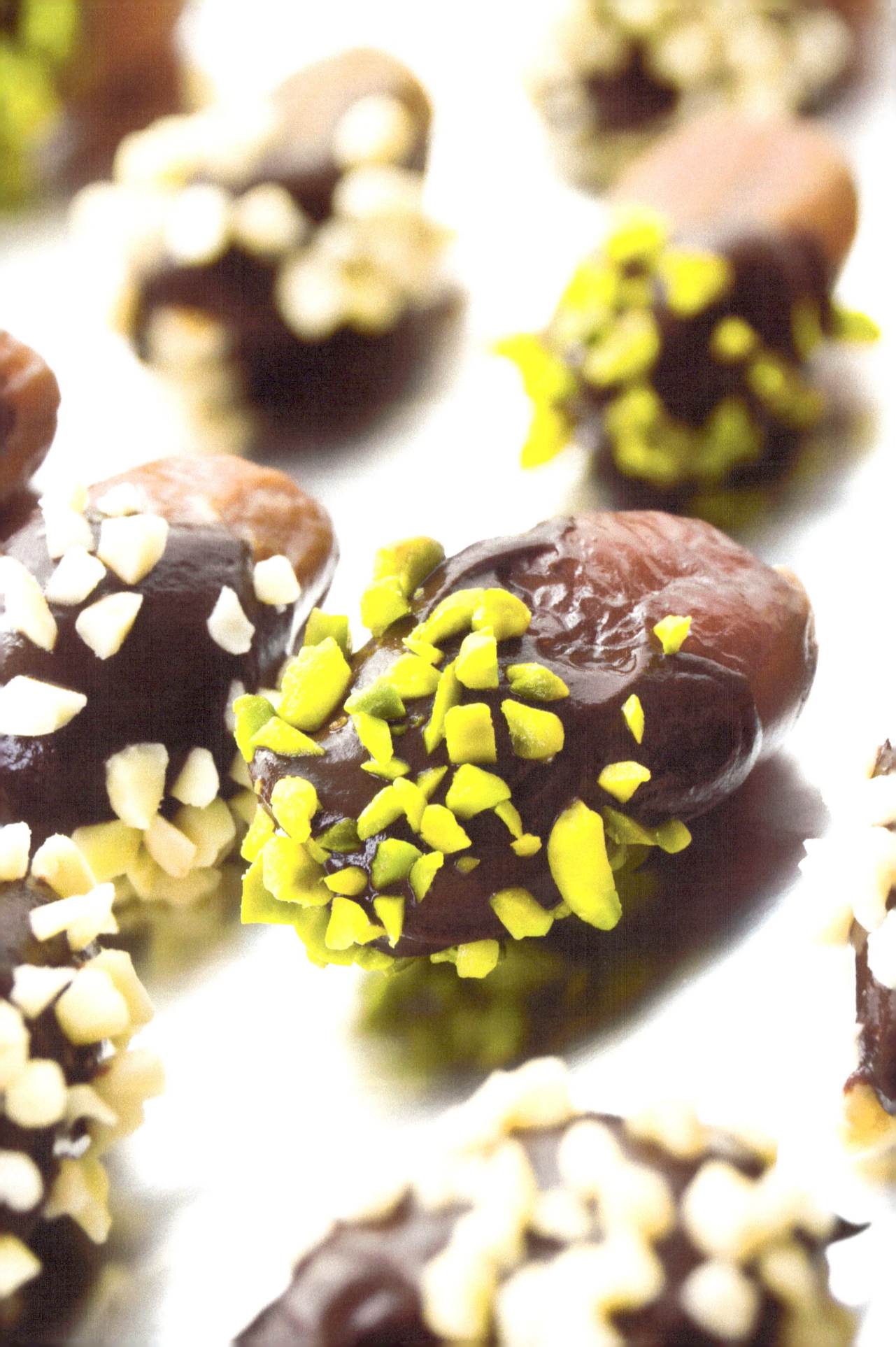

CHOCOLATE COVERED DATES

INGREDIENTS

- 1 pack pitted dates
- ¼ cup sunflower seed butter
- ½ cup unsalted cashews
- 2 tbsp condensed coconut milk
- 4 tbsp tahini
- 2 tbsp shaved roasted cocoa nibs

INSTRUCTIONS

1. Place the dates on parchment paper and make a small slit down the middle.
2. Fill half the dates with tahini and the other half with sunflower seed better.
3. Then add the cashews and drizzle with condensed coconut milk.
4. Shave the roasted cocoa nibs.

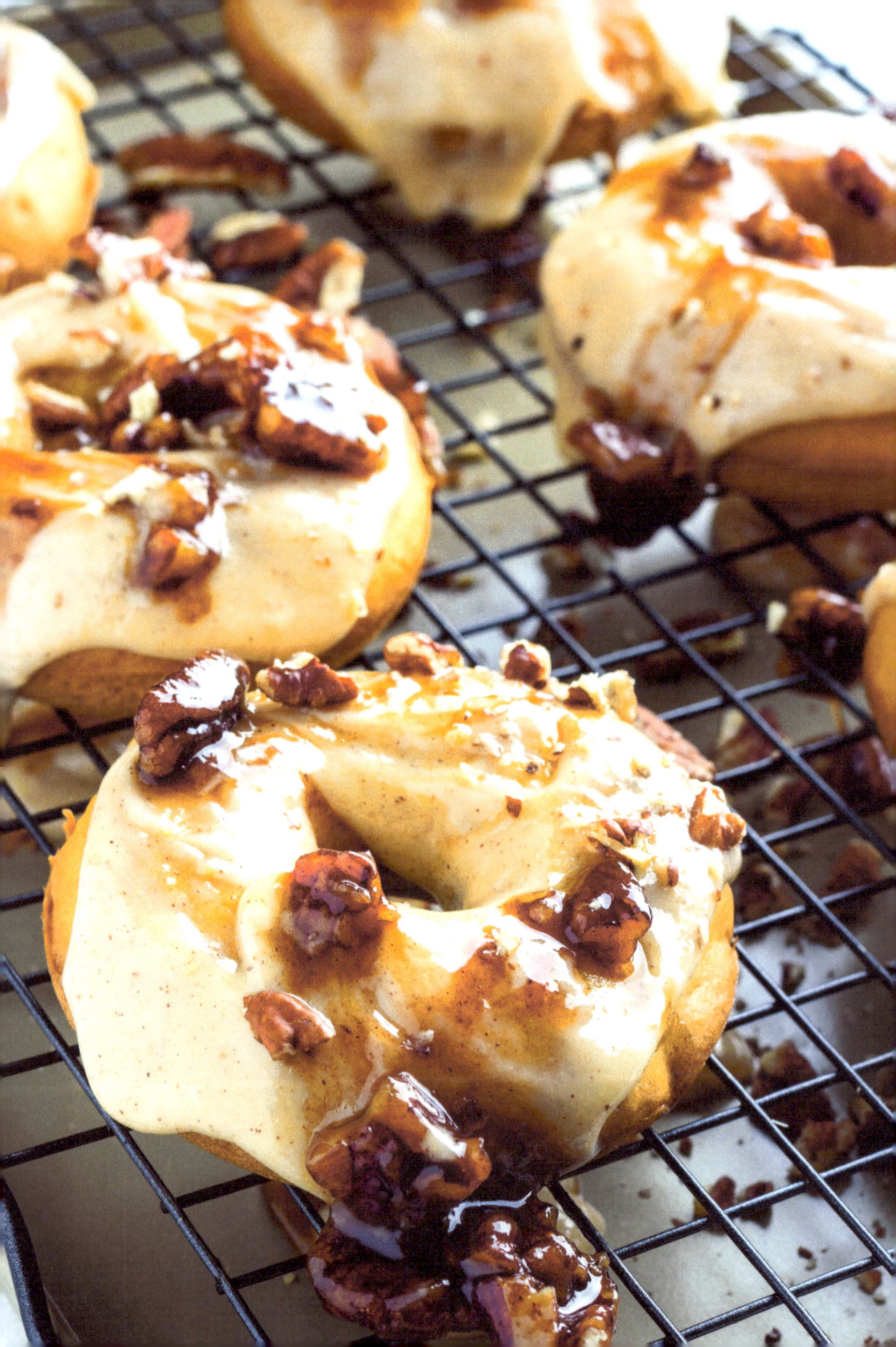

CANDIED PECAN MAPLE SYRUP DONUTS

INGREDIENTS

- 1 ¼ cups milk, I used Not Milk
- ½ cup melted butter
- ½ maple syrup
- ½ cup brown sugar
- 2 tsp vanilla
- 1 tsp baking powder
- 1 tbsp cinnamon
- ¼ tsp salt
- 2 ½ cups unbleached all-purpose flour
- 1 tbsp cardamom

Maple Glaze
- 2 tbsp maple syrup
- 2 tbsp milk
- 2 tbsp melted butter
- ½ cup powdered sugar

Cinnamon Cream Cheese Frosting
- 1 ¼ cups powdered sugar
- ¼ cup cream cheese
- 6 tbsp softened butter
- 1 tsp cinnamon
- 1 tbsp tahini
- ½ tbsp cardamom

Toasted Maple Pecan
- 1 tbsp plant-based butter
- 2 tbsp maple syrup
- ½ cup chopped pecan

INSTRUCTIONS

1. Preheat the oven to 350° Fahrenheit.
2. Mix the almond milk, melted butter, maple syrup, vanilla, cinnamon, baking powder, cardamom, and baking soda together. Then add the flour and mix until a thick batter is formed.
3. Using a ⅓ measuring cup, spoon the batter into donut silicone molds that have been greased with butter. Be careful not to overfill the molds. Bake for 20-25 minutes or until the donuts have risen.
4. While the donuts are baking, whisk together the maple glaze ingredients in a bowl. Once the donuts are done baking, remove them from the bran and allow them to cool for two minutes. Coat each donut with the maple glaze before serving.
5. Heat a small skillet, add the pecans, and toast for 2-5 minutes, or until the aroma is fragrant. Add the butter and maple syrup and cook for about 2 minutes, or until the syrup is bubbling and thick. Allow the pecans to cool before sprinkling them on top of the donuts.

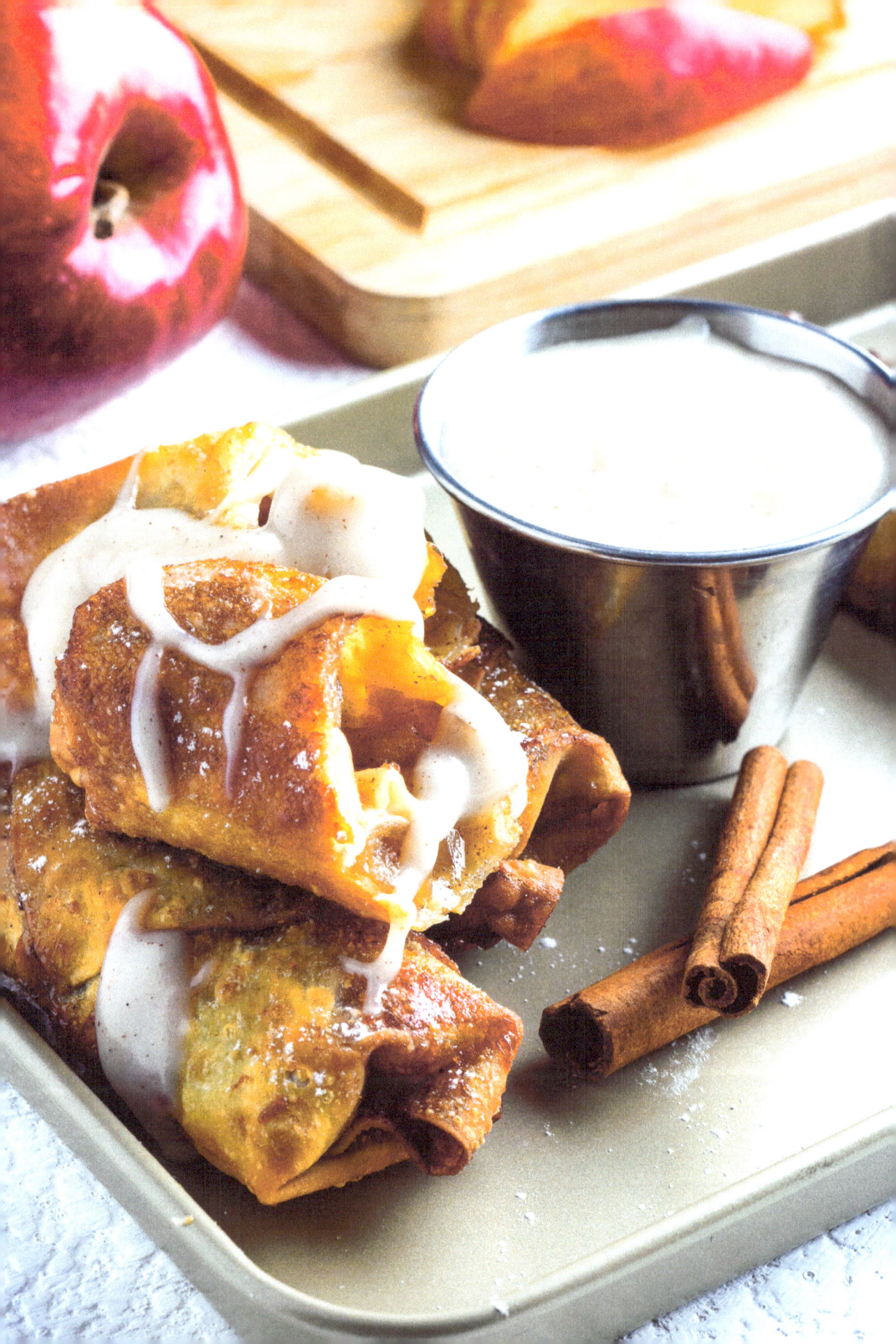

APPLE PIE EGGROLLS

INGREDIENTS

- 1 bag of apples
- 2 tbsp softened butter
- ½ cup light brown sugar
- ¼ c cinnamon
- 2 tbsp cardamom
- ¼ cup water
- ½ tsp nutmeg
- ½ tsp all spice
- 1 pack of Vegan Egg Roll Wraps
- Grapeseed oil

Cream Cheese Frosting

- 4 tbsp brown sugar
- 1 tsp vanilla
- 2 tbsp lemon juice
- 4 oz plain cream cheese

INSTRUCTIONS

1. Wash the apples, peel them, and dice them into ¼ inch pieces. Set aside.
2. In a small pot on medium low heat, add butter, cinnamon, cardamom, nutmeg, brown sugar, and all spice. Cook until a thick consistency forms. Stir occasionally and keep the heat low to avoid burning. Remove the sauce from the heat once it has thickened.
3. In a medium pot, add water. When water comes to a boil, add apples.
4. Cook the apples for 30-45 minutes, or until tender. Set it aside after removing from heat and let apples cool.
5. Add the sauce to the apples and stir well to coat each apple. If the sauce isn't thick enough, add more sugar and cook 5-10 minutes.
6. Once apples cool add two to four tablespoons to egg roll wrap. Fold each wrap and set to the side.
7. Once all are folded drop in fryer.
8. Cook for 2-3 minutes or until golden brown.
9. Place eggrolls on cooling rack to drain excess oil.

If using a deep fryer, please follow instructions for oil. If using a cast iron skillet, use 1-2 cups of grapeseed oil.

PECAN CHOCOLATE CHIP COOKIES

Cookies are always a win. I love a crisp on the edge, soft on the inside cookie with lots of unexpected hints of spices. This cookie is the best cookie I have ever had. It took me about five years to perfect this recipe as well (Mac and cheese story). If you are not a fan of pecans, omit them and enjoy the perfect chocolate chip cookie.

INGREDIENTS

- 1 ¼ c brown sugar
- ½ c butter softened
- ½ tsp cinnamon
- 1 tbsp tahini
- 2 tsp cornstarch
- 1 ½ c unbleached flour
- ½ c chopped pecans
- ½ tsp cardamom
- 1 tbsp ground flaxseed
- 2 tsp vanilla extract
- 1 ¼ c chocolate chips
- ¼ tsp sea salt
- 1 tsp baking soda
- 2 ½ tbsp water
- *Omit pecan for a delicious chocolate chip cookie*

INSTRUCTIONS

1. Pre-heat oven to 350° Farenheit. Place cookies on foil or line cookie sheet with parchment paper.
2. Mix the ground flaxseed and water in a small bowl and set aside to make your flax egg.
3. In a large bowl using a whisk beat the butter and brown sugar for 1-2 minutes until creamy.
4. Add the vanilla, flax egg, tahini, cinnamon and cardamom and mix to combine.
5. Next, add the flour Sprinkle cornstarch, baking soda and salt on top of the flour. Whisk until combined.
6. Add in the chocolate chips to incorporate by hand.
7. Use ⅓ measuring cup, roll dough into balls using ⅓ measuring cup. Place on the foil and bake for 10 minutes. Pull the cookies out, flatten them with a wooden spatula and bake for two minutes. Do not over bake (if so, crumble and use it as a dessert or smoothie topping).
8. Let cool on the cookie sheet for five minutes, then transfer to a cooling rack. The cookies will firm up as they cool.

SUNFLOWER SEED BUTTER COOKIES

Sunflower butter because that's my business in my Tabitha Brown voice! Why not? This cookie is one of those do not it until you try it. This is a peanut butter times 1000, next level deliciousness. So soft and chewy, you will forget about peanut butter.

INGREDIENTS

- 1 ¼ cup brown sugar
- 1 tbsp sunflower seed butter
- ½ tsp cardamom
- 1 tbsp ground flaxseed
- 2 tsp vanilla extract
- 1 ½ c unbleached flour
- ¼ tsp sea salt
- 1 tsp baking soda
- 2 ½ tbsp water
- ½ cup butter softened
- ½ tsp cinnamon
- 1 tbsp tahini
- 2 tsp cornstarch

INSTRUCTIONS

1. Pre heat oven to 350°. Place cookies on foil or line cookie sheet with parchment paper.
2. Mix the ground flaxseed and water in a small bowl and set aside to make your flax egg.
3. In a large bowl using a whisk beat the butter and brown sugar for 1-2 minutes until creamy.
4. Add the vanilla, flax egg, tahini, sunflower seed butter, cinnamon and cardamom and mix to combine.
5. Next, add the flour Sprinkle cornstarch, baking soda and salt on top of the flour. Whisk until combined.
6. Use ⅓ measuring cup, roll dough into balls using ⅓ measuring cup. Place on the foil and bake for 10 minutes. Pull the cookies out, flatten them with a wooden spatula and bake for two minutes. Do not over bake (if so, crumble and use it as a dessert or smoothie topping).
7. Let cool on the cookie sheet for five minutes, then transfer to a cooling rack. The cookies will firm up as they cool.
8. Serve warm or cool. Enjoy!

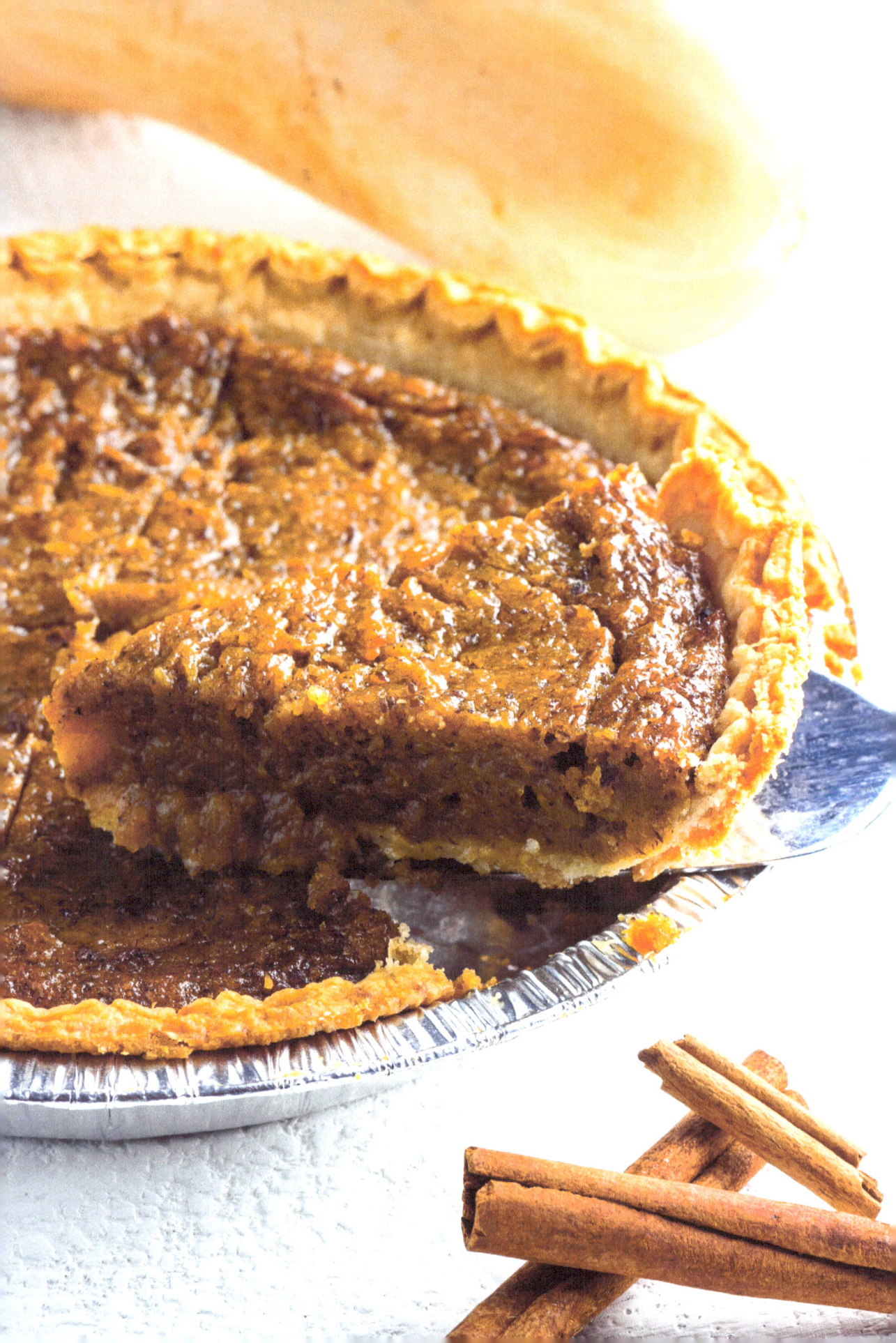

CANDIED BUTTERNUT SQUASH PIE

I absolutely love butternut squash! It is another versatile vegetable that will taste like anything you season it to be. I've made curry squash, another favorite for another cookbook. Squash has far better benefits than sweet potatoes and once I learned the pro and cons of both I substitute this for recipe requiring sweet potatoes. What's a family gathering without sweet potato pie? Not one to remember right? The only difference is removing dairy.

INGREDIENTS

- 1 large Butternut Squash
- ½ cup brown sugar
- ⅛ tsp cardamom
- 2 tbsp butter
- 4 tbsp water
- 1 tbsp cinnamon
- 1 tsp vanilla
- 1 tsp nutmeg
- 2 tbsp ground flax seed
- 2 Pie crust

INSTRUCTIONS

1. Preheat oven to 400° Fahrenheit.
2. Place squash in the oven for 20-30 minutes or until knife glides through. This will allow you to -cut the squash easier and decrease cooking time.
3. Mix flax seed and water in small cup and set aside.
4. Remove from oven and let cool.
5. Once cooled remove the top stem and bottom, remove the skin and slice into ¼ inch pieces.
6. Transfer squash to a bowl, add flax "egg" and mix with whisk or cake mixer.
7. In a small skillet on medium low add cinnamon, brown sugar, cane sugar, vanilla, cardamom, and nutmeg. Stir until blended and smooth consistency.
8. Add more sugar and spices according to taste.
9. Transfer to a pie shell. Place in oven.
10. Cook according to pie shell instructions.
11. Let cool and serve.

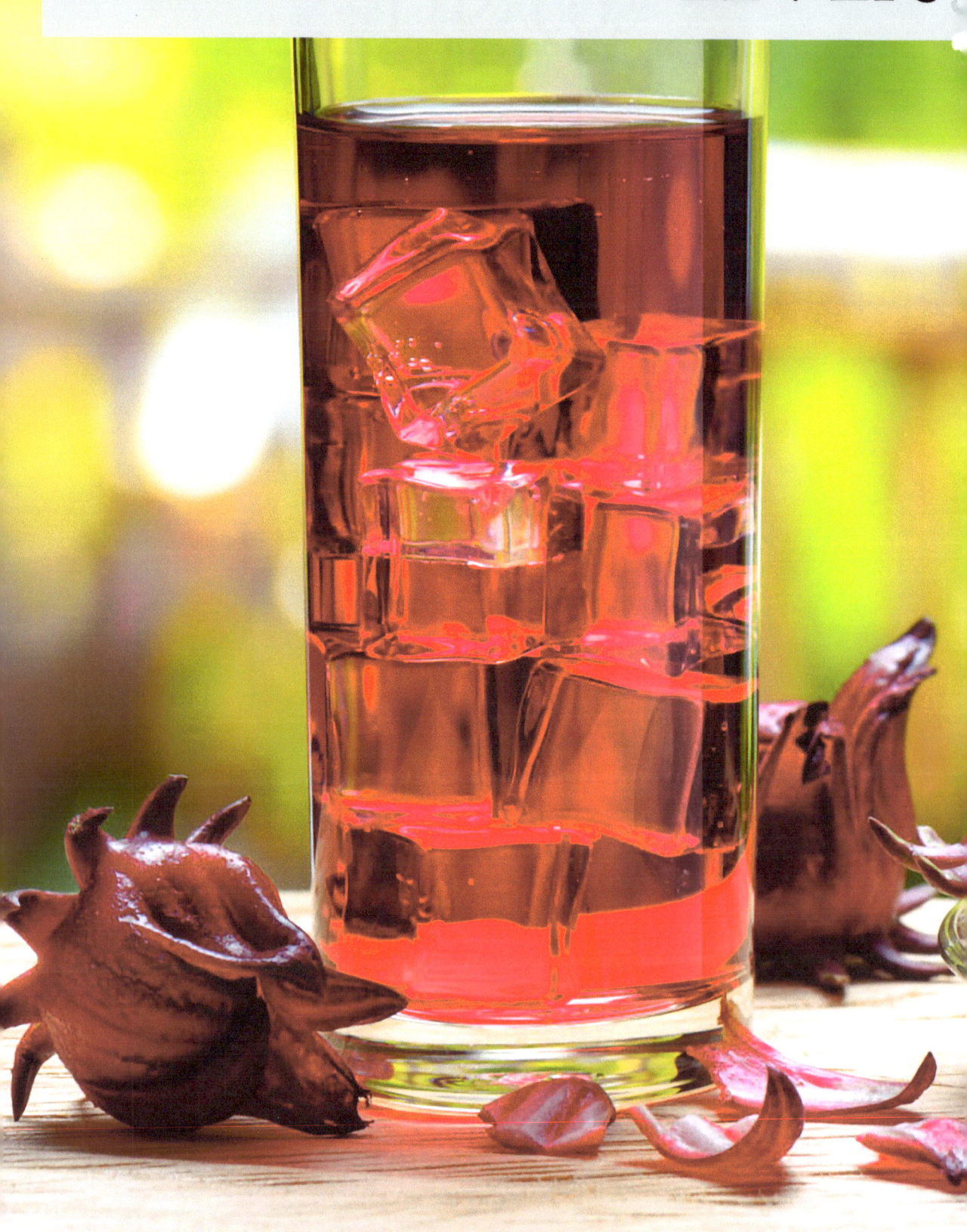

BEVER

AGES

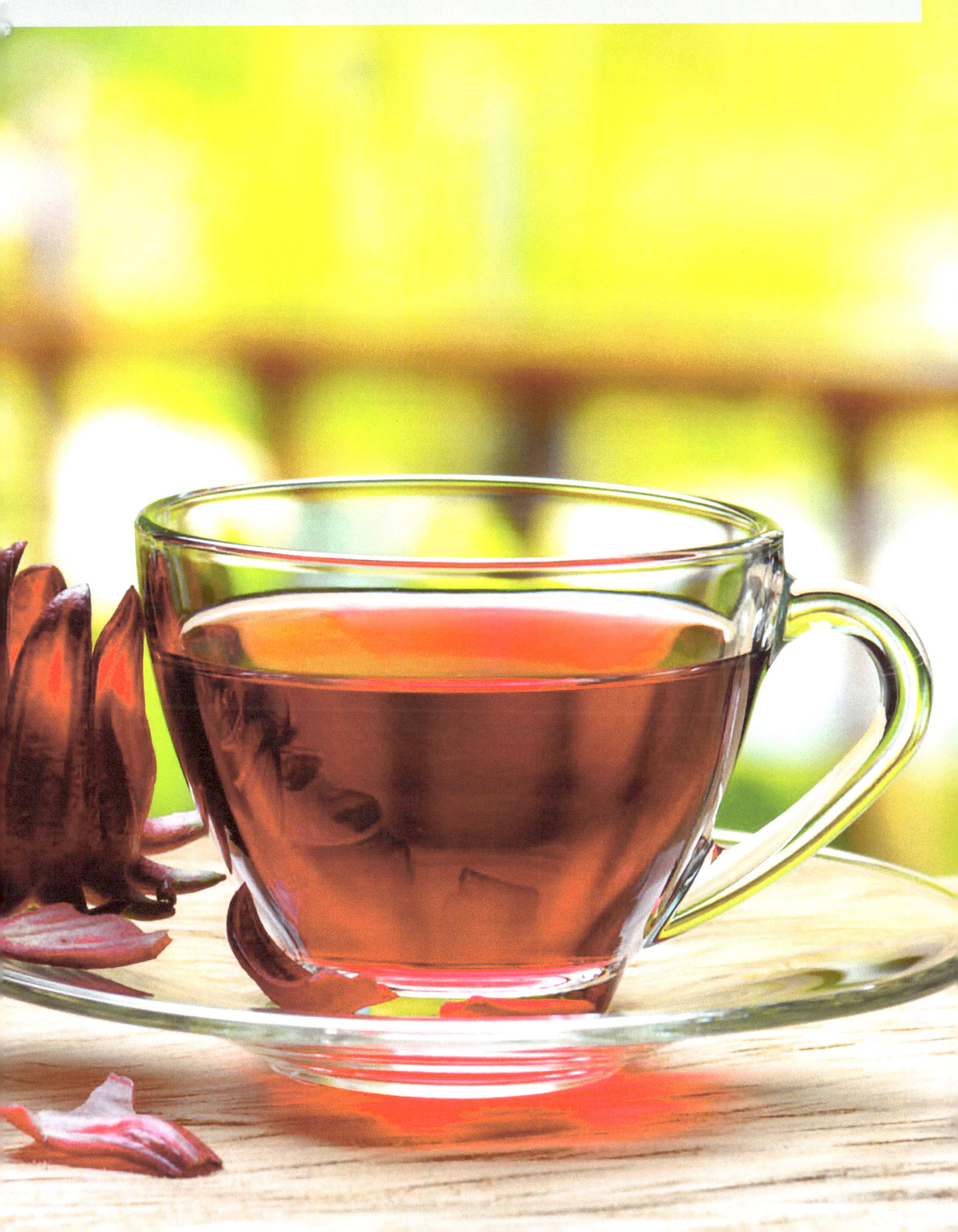

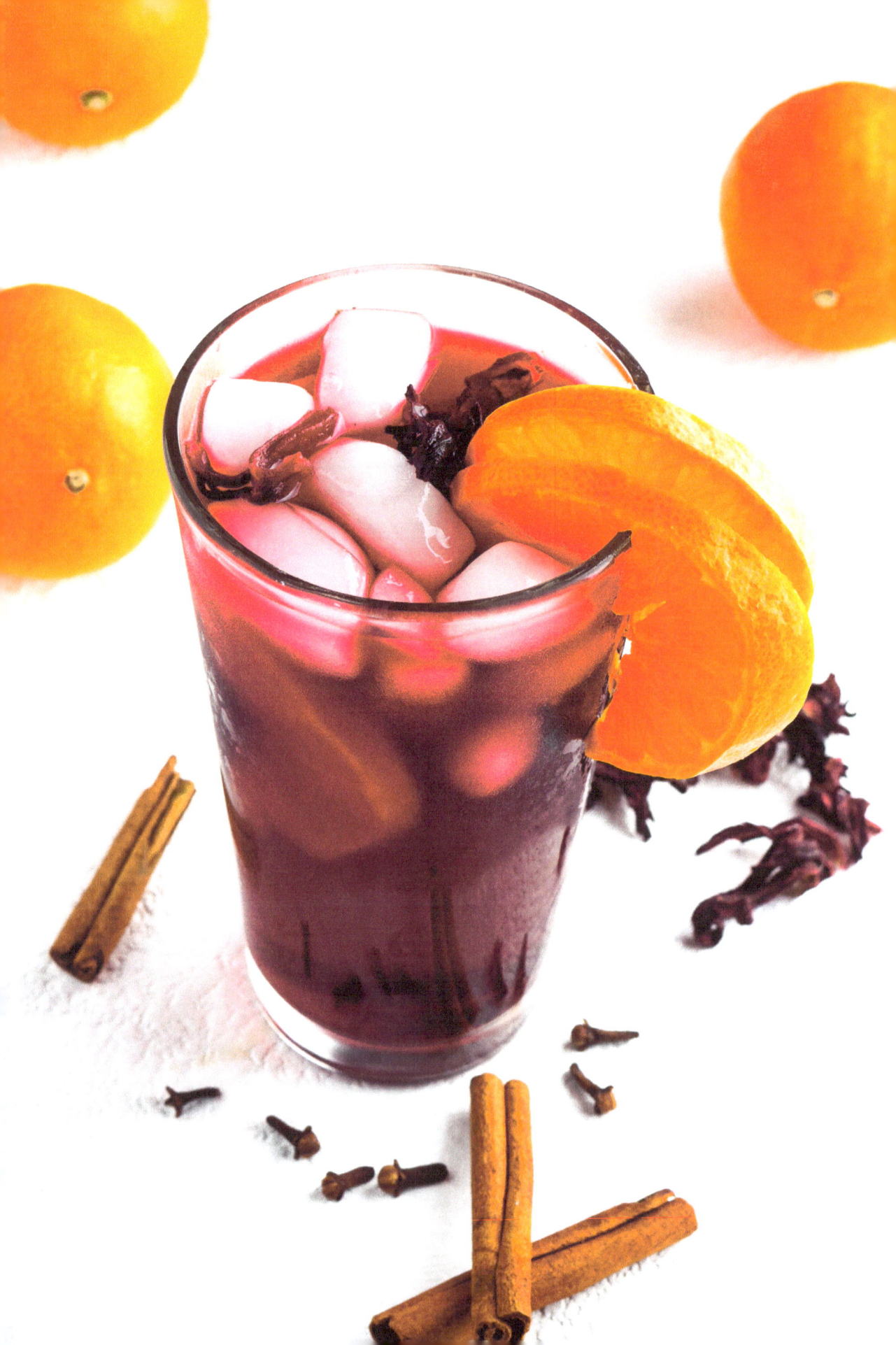

SORREL TEA

INGREDIENTS

- 1 ½ cups dried sorrel petals
- 9 cups of spring water
- 3 small cinnamon sticks
- 1 orange peeled
- 4 cloves
- ½ tbsp ground allspice
- Thumb of ginger chopped
- Maple syrup

INSTRUCTIONS

1. Gather a small pitcher and fill it with the water. Cut the ginger into small slices and add to pitcher with cinnamon sticks, orange pieces, allspice, and cloves.
2. Cover the pitcher and let steep for up to five hours or overnight.
3. Pour the sorrel mixture into a sieve and allow it to strain into another bowl.
4. Set aside the sorrel pieces for another recipe.
5. Sweeten to your taste by adding the maple syrup to the mixture.
6. Refrigerate to chill

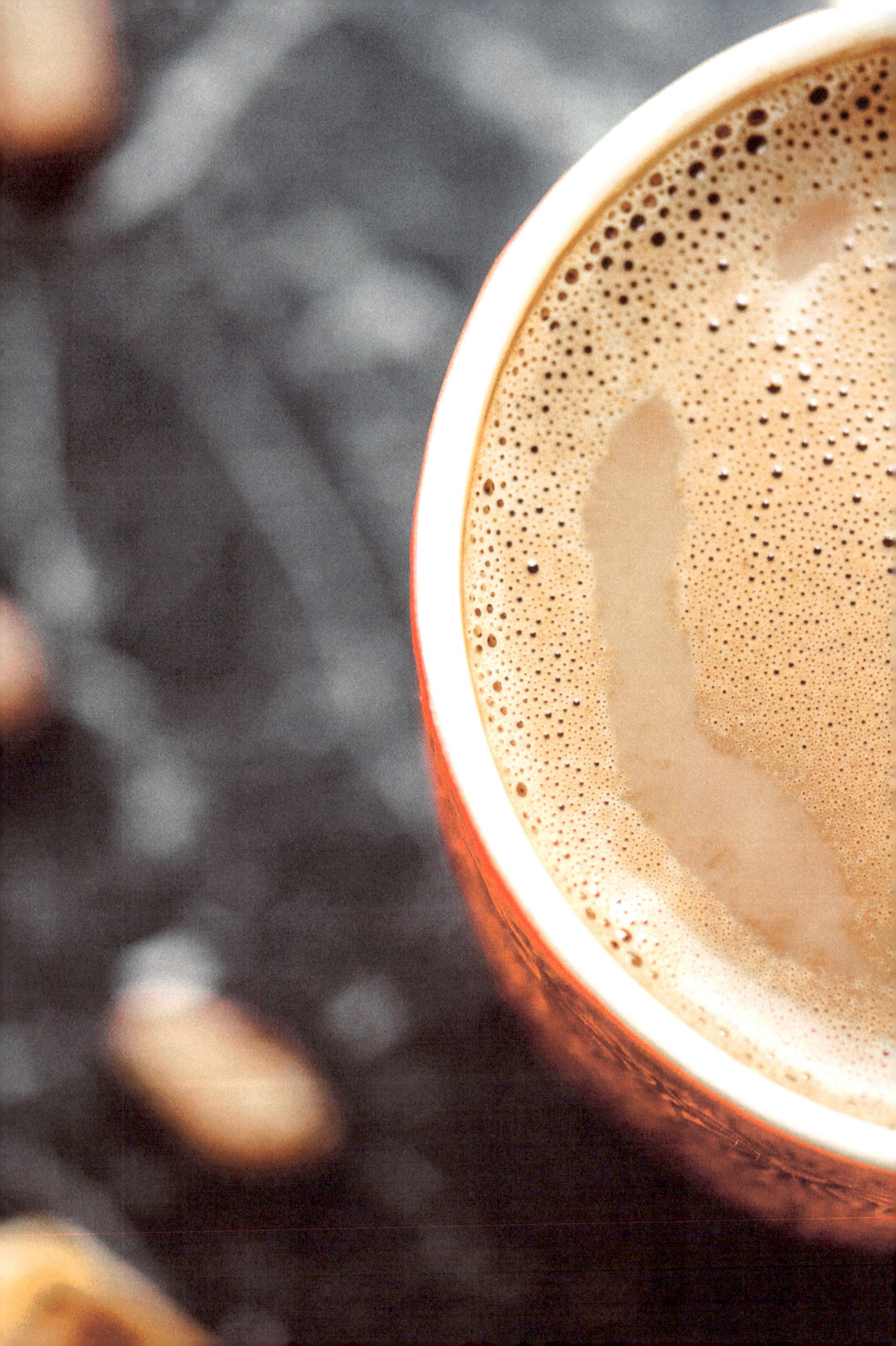

HOT COCOA

INGREDIENTS

- 2 c spring water
- ½ c grated cocoa
- 2 cups water
- 1 cup plant-based milk
- ¼ cup plant-based coconut Condensed milk
- Maple syrup to taste
- 1 tbsp vanilla extract
- 3 Cinnamon sticks
- 4 Star Anise

INSTRUCTIONS

1. Pour water into a saucepan and boil over medium heat for five minutes. Add cinnamon sticks, star anise, and cocoa to the boiling water. Boil for 15 minutes, or until the cocoa is melted. Take off the heat and strain.
2. Return the pot to a low medium heat and stir in the milk, maple syrup, and condensed milk.

STRAWBERRY LIMEADE

INGREDIENTS

- 8 cups of spring water
- 1 container of strawberries
- 4 key limes
- ½ cup maple syrup

INSTRUCTIONS

1. Wash strawberries with water and white distilled vinegar. Take 12 of the strawberries and remove the tops. In a bowl, smash them with a fork and set aside.
2. Lime and strawberry juice Mix well and add maple syrup.
3. Pour water into the pitcher, then add the strawberry mix and stir.
4. Add more sweetener if desired.

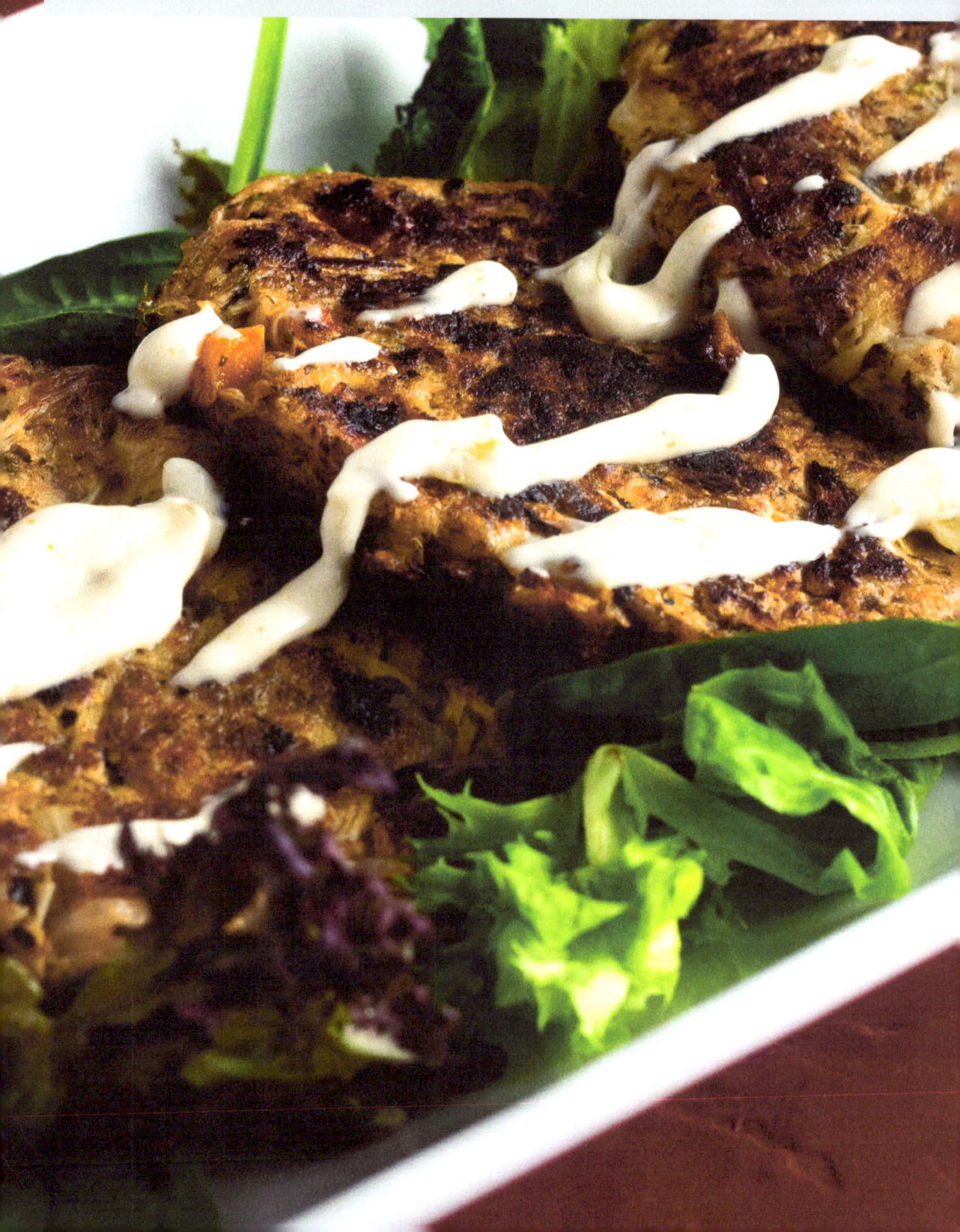

BON

US

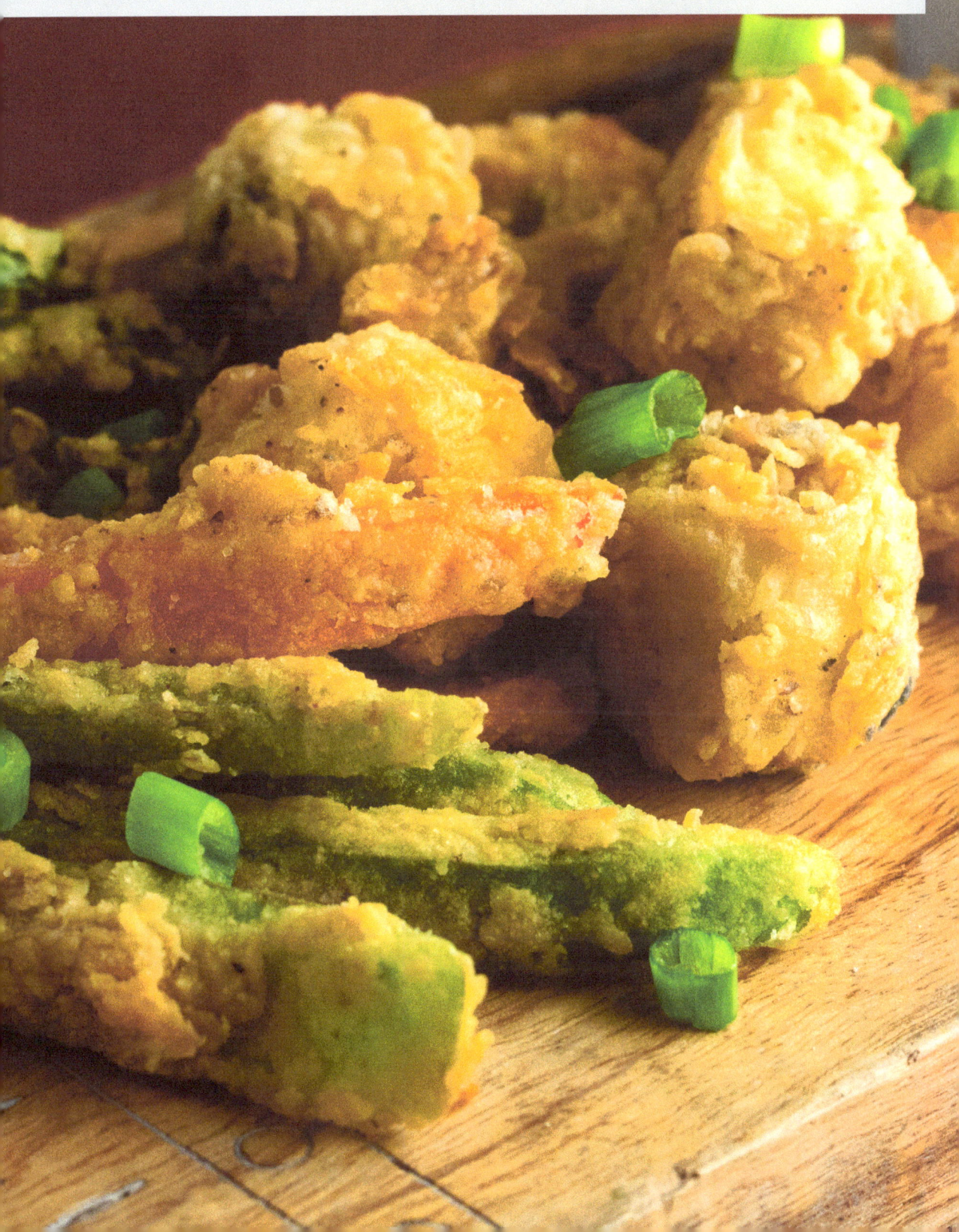

SEEFOOD LOVERS!!! ALTERNATIVES TO YOUR FAVORITES!

The traditional holidays meals have changed for some over the years for many reasons. Some people want something different or may have food restrictions. We know that seafood has become a popular request for any occasion i.e., holidays, celebrations, etc. Many people struggle releasing these foods when going plant based. I know how important it is to satisfy the pallet, these next few recipes will allow you to get creative in the kitchen, have fun, and realize plant-based food does not miss a beat.

I read a post earlier this year of someone asking if there is a such thing as a plant-based pescatarian. I immediately chuckled because I have Seefood Saturday very often and these dishes do not miss a beat. I understand how much people love seafood and I wanted to create dishes that satisfied these nostalgic moments. When you truly realize the connection between what you put in your body and your overall health you will begin to make changes for the betterment of you life.

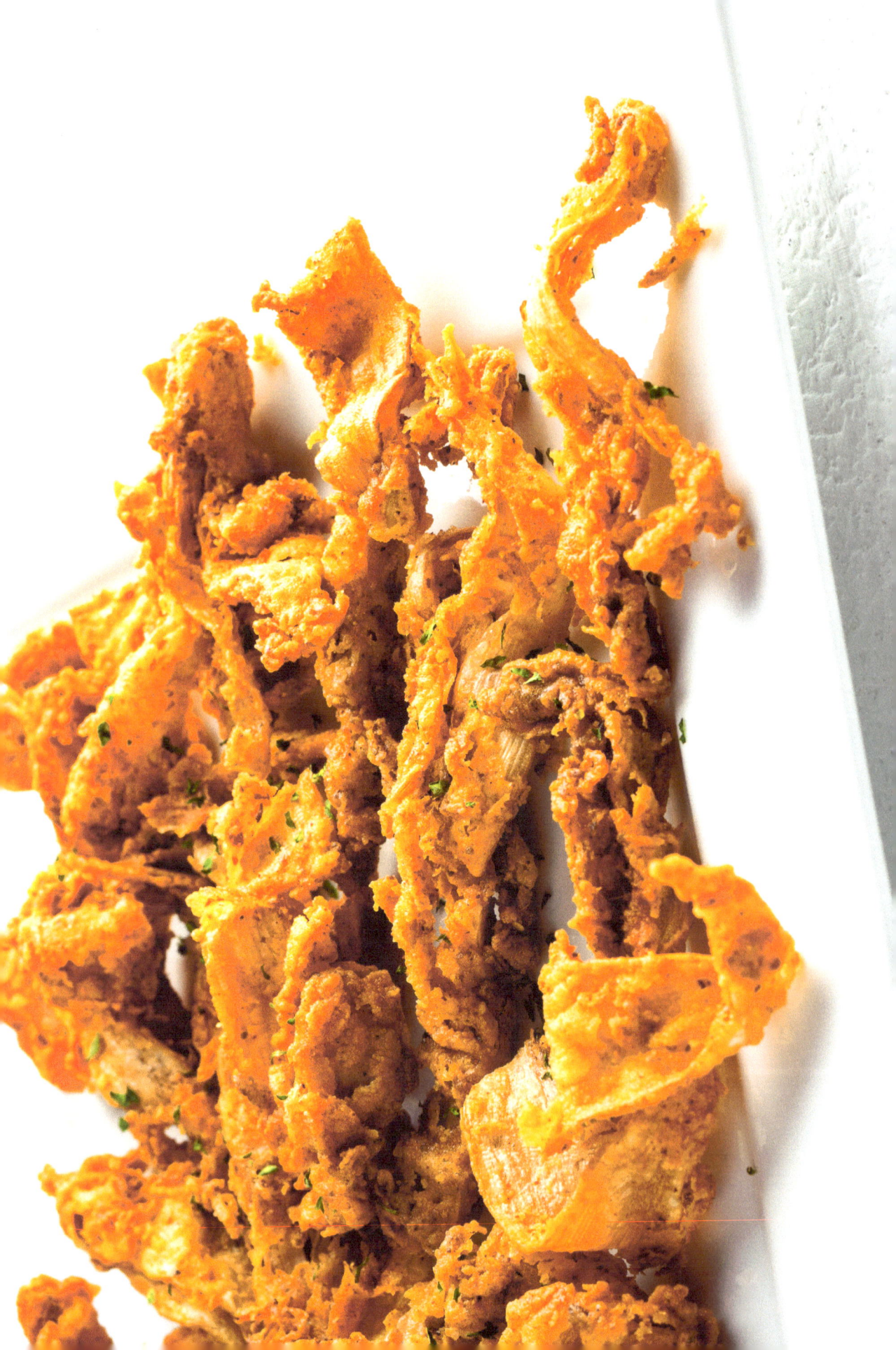

PHISH

INGREDIENTS

- 2 cans of banana blossom
- ¼ cup crushed seaweed sheets
- 1 tbs Old Bay Seasoning (optional)
- ½ tbs ground black pepper
- 1 tbsp kelp flakes
- 1 tbsp dulse flakes
- 1 bag of fish fry seasoning
- 2 cups corn meal
- 2 tbsp flax seed
- ½ cup plant- based unsweetened milk
- *Grapeseed oil**

INSTRUCTIONS

1. Drain water from both cans of banana blossom and place them in a bowl. Add half of seaweed flakes, old bay, kelp, and dulse flakes. Marinate for at least four hours.
2. Remove banana blossom from refrigerator.
3. In a bowl add flax seeds and milk and set aside.
4. In a bowl add garbanzo flour with spices and other bowl add the corn meal with spices.
5. Turn deep fryer to 340º Fahrenheit. Test oil heat by sprinkling flour.
6. Dip banana blossom in wet batter, then fish fry batter flour, then wet batter, then dip in corn meal.
7. Remove banana blossoms from grease and place on paper towel or cooling rack to drain grease.
8. Garnish with parsley and serve with hom

*If you are using a deep fryer, please follow instructions for oil. If you are using a cast iron skillet, use one to two cups of grapeseed oil.

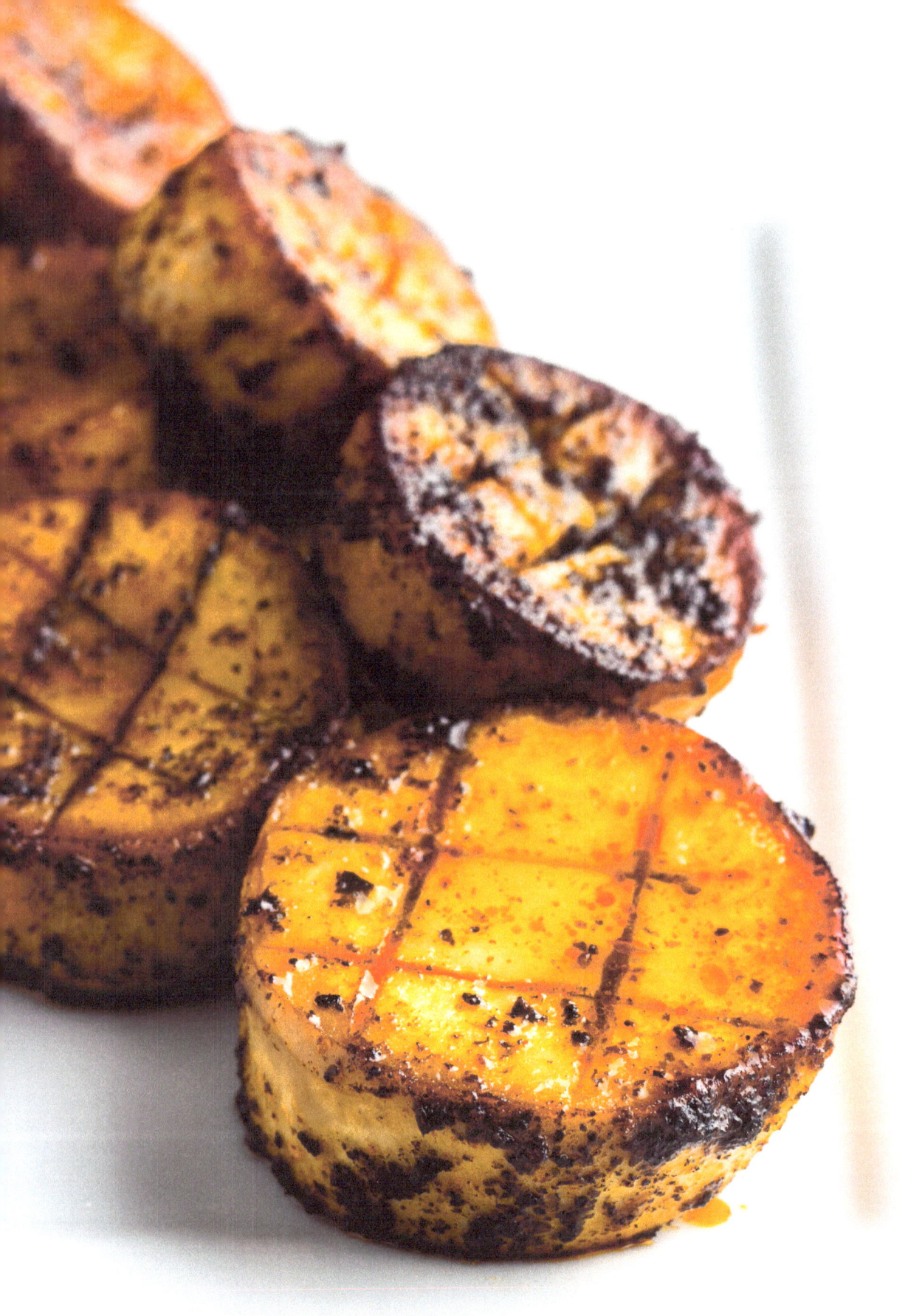

SCALLOPS

INGREDIENTS

- 2 pack of large oyster mushrooms
- ¼ cup crushed seaweed sheets
- 1 tbs Old Bay Seasoning (optional)
- ½ tbs ground black pepper
- 1 tbsp kelp flakes
- 1 tbsp dulse flakes
- 1 tbsp grape seed oil (optional)

INSTRUCTIONS

1. Wash mushrooms very well and let them dry on a paper towel.
2. Mushrooms should be dry. Cut the top off, then slice them ¼ inch thick.
3. Score them diagonal across both sides.
4. Add half of seaweed flakes, old bay, kelp, and dulse flakes. Marinate for at least 4 hours or overnight.
5. Heat a medium saucepan on medium heat, when hot add king oyster mushrooms and sear each side 3-5 minutes.
6. Garnish with parsley and serve with homemade tartar or sriracha aioli.

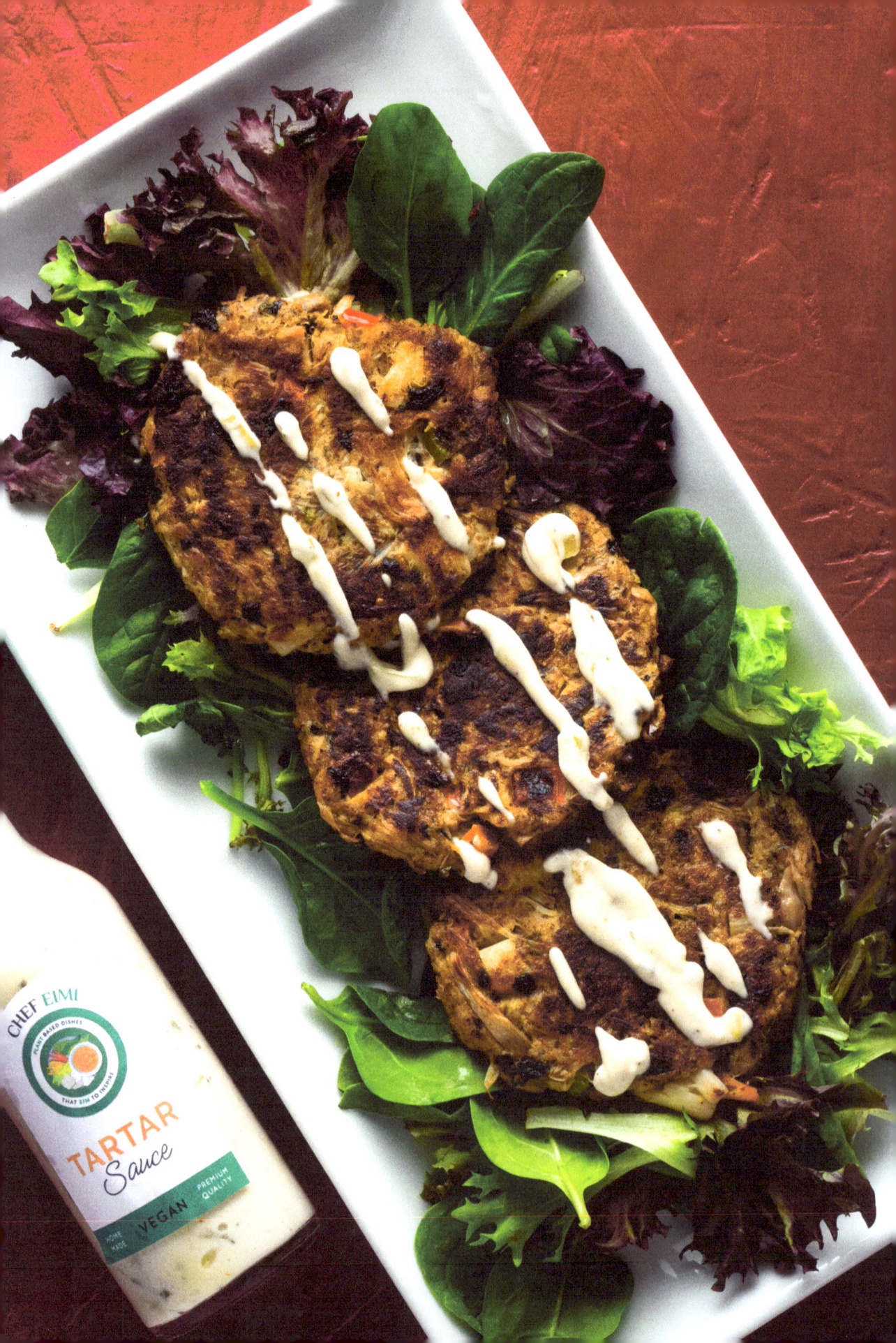

JOYCE KRAB CAKES

I'm sure you're wondering what Joyce Cakes are!! Well, these are my version of crab cakes, named after my aunt Joyce, who lived in Maryland. Therefore, since Maryland is known for crabs (specifically blue crabs), it made sense to correlate the dish with my amazing aunt. I did not have the opportunity to meet her before she transcended, but we spoke over the phone several times and she always told me how proud of me she was, and this was before I started my plant-based journey. I know each time I make this dish, she is with me in spirit and guiding me.

INGREDIENTS

- 1 can of Jackfruit in Brine
- 1 cup Nori Flakes (Seaweed Flakes)
- 2 tbsp. Dulse Flakes
- 3 tbsp. Old Bay Seasoning
- 2 tbsp Red Pepper (diced)
- 1 tbsp. Seasoning Salt
- 2 tbsp. Onion Powder
- ¼ cup garbanzo Flour
- ¼ cup grapeseed Oil
- Pinch of black pepper
- 2 tbsp. Kelp Flakes
- *2 cups Breadcrumbs (Homemade and optional)
- ¼ cup red onion
- (diced) 2 tbsp Green Pepper (diced)
- 2 tbsp. Paprika
- 1 tbsp. Smoked Paprika
- 2 tbsp Sea Salt or Celtic Salt
- *Flax Egg (1 tbsp. ground flax, 2 tbsp. water) or bowl of water
- 1 can of Palm of Artichoke Heart (the inside soft part only)

INSTRUCTIONS

1. Drain jackfruit, remove any seeds, then cut the ends (hard) part off. Soak for at least four hours or overnight in water. This removes the sticky residue.

2. Drain and dry very well, jackfruit holds a lot of water. Season jackfruit with nori flakes, dulse flakes, old base seasoning, paprika, smoked paprika, and onion powder. Marinate for at least four hours or overnight.

3. Be sure all the liquid is removed from the seasoned jackfruit, add the palm of heart artichoke, flax egg, onion, garbanzo flour red, green, and yellow peppers.

4. Heat cast-iron skillet on medium-high heat, add grapeseed oil and form patties.

5. If you like the crispy outside coat Joyce cakes with breadcrumbs if not add patties to oil.

6. Cook each side for two to three minutes or until golden brown.

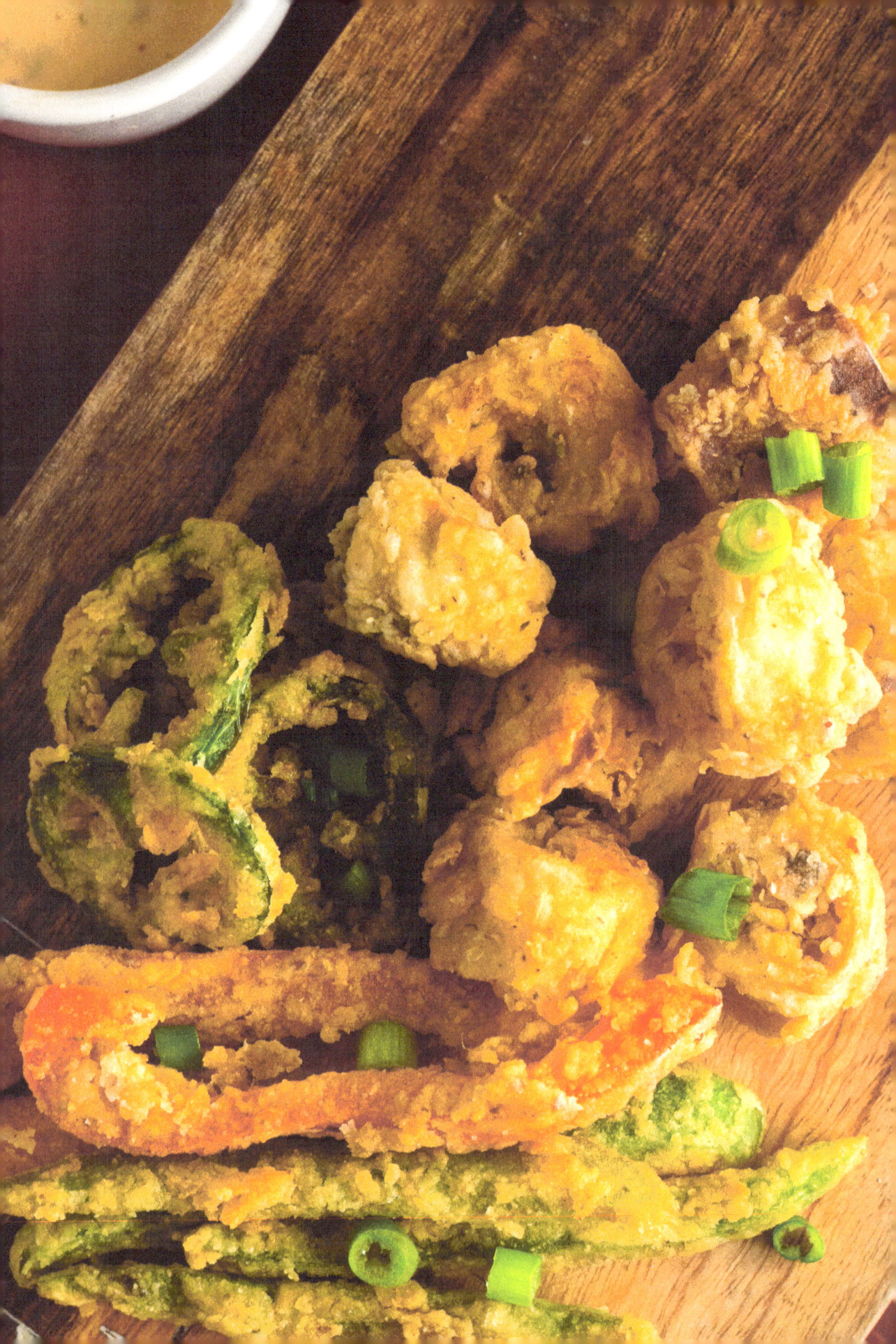

CALAMARI

INGREDIENTS

- 1 can of Whole Artichoke Hearts or Salad Cut
- 2 tbsp. Dulse Flakes
- **2 cups Breadcrumbs (Homemade)
- 1 tbsp. Seasoning Salt
- 1 tbsp. Onion Powder
- Pinch of Pepper
- Scallions (optional)
- ¼ c Nori Flakes (Seaweed Flakes)
- 2 c Unbleached Flour
- 3 tbsp. Old Bay Seasoning
- 2 tbsp. Paprika
- 1 tbsp. Smoked Paprika
- *Grapeseed Oil
- Flax Egg (1 tbsp. ground flax, 2 tbsp. water) or bowl of water

INSTRUCTIONS

1. If a whole can of artichoke is used, slice artichokes about 1-2 inches thick, if salad cut is used, they are already sliced perfectly.
2. Remove inside "meat" (not sure what to call it). This is used for Joyce cakes in the next recipe.
3. Add all seasoning and marinate for at least four hours or overnight.
4. *Prepare the flax egg. Let the flax "egg" sit for at least 10 mins.
5. Season Flour with Old Bay, seasoning salt, onion powder, pepper, and dulse flakes.
6. Season flax egg with paprika and smoked paprika.
7. Dip calamari in wet batter, then flour, wet batter, and breadcrumbs. Fry until crispy.

**Save your old bread and the end pieces, toast, and blend.

****** Peppers and jalapenos for presentation only. If you love tempura veggies, add them. Use the same process as above but do not use the same batter unless you do not mind the seafood taste.

CHICKPEA SALAD

INGREDIENTS

- 2 oz cans of chickpeas
- 2 tbsp finely diced red onion
- ¼ cup crushed seaweed sheets
- 1 tbs Old Bay Seasoning (optional)
- ½ cup soy free plant-based mayo
- ⅛ tsp black salt
- 1 tbsp celery seeds
- ½ tbs ground black pepper
- 1 tbsp kelp flakes
- 1 tbsp dulse flakes
- ½ tsp smoked paprika

INSTRUCTIONS

1. Drain the water from both cans of chickpeas, rinse and set aside.
2. In a medium bowl smash the chickpeas with a potato masher, leave some who pieces for texture.
3. After you have smashed the chickpeas to desired consistency add all ingredients and mix well.
4. Garnish with smoked paprika. Place in refrigerator to chill for one to two hours or serve as is with crackers.

SKRIMP

INGREDIENTS

- 2 pack of large king oyster mushrooms
- ¼ cup crushed seaweed sheets
- 1 tbs Old Bay Seasoning (optional)
- ½ tbs ground black pepper
- 1 tbsp kelp flakes
- 1 tbsp dulse flakes
- *Grapeseed oil

INSTRUCTIONS

1. Wash mushrooms very well and let the dry on a paper towel.
2. Mushrooms should be dry. Cut the top off, then slice them ¼ inch thick. Use a bottle top to make a whole then cut a ½ inch opening.
3. Add seaweed flakes, old bay, kelp, and dulse flakes. Marinate for at least 4 hours or overnight.
4. Turn deep fryer to 340^0 Fahrenheit..
5. In a bowl add flax seeds and plant-based milk and set aside.
6. In a bowl add garbanzo flour with spices and other bowl add the corn meal with spices.
7. Dip king oyster mushrooms in wet batter, then fish fry batter flour, then wet batter, then dip in corn meal.
8. Test temperature by sprinkling flour into oil. Cook for 3-5 minutes or until crispy.
9. Remove from grease and place on paper towel or cooling rack to drain oil.

INDEX

A
- All purpose
- Apple

B
- Banana Blossom
- Barbecue
- Bake
- Baking
- Balsamic
- Bean
- Green
- Broth
- Brown sugar
- Bonus
- Bundt Cake
- Butter
- Butternut squash

C
- Cabbage, red
- Cake
- Carrots
- Cardamom
- Cauliflower
- Cheese
- Chiai
- Chickpeas
- Chocolate, chip
- Cloves
- Cinnamon
- Coconut, milk
- Coconut amino

- Cream cheese
- Cucumber
- Cumin

D
- Dill Distilled Vinegar
- Dulse Flakes

F
- Flax
- Flour,
- All Purpose
- Garbanzo

G
- Garbanzo, Flour
- Garlic
- Grapeseed
- Green Bean

J
- Jackfruit
- Jalapeños

K
- Kelp Flakes
- King Oyster Mushroom

L
- Lemon
- Liquid Smoke
- Liquid Amino

M
- Macaroni
- Maple

INDEX

- Meatloaf
- Mashed, red potato
- Milk
- Mushroom

N
- Nuts
- NutmegO
- Onion powder
- Old Bay
- Oyster Mushroom

P
- Paprika
- Phish
- Plant-based
- Potato
- Pot Roast
- Purple Cabbage
- Purple Onion

Q
- Quinoa

R
- Red Bell Pepper
- Red Potato
- Rosemary

S
- Salt
- Seasoning Salt
- Scrimp
- Smoked Paprika
- Sorrel
- Soy
- Squash
- "Steak"

T
- Tahini

U
- umami

V
- Vegie Broth

W
- Walnut
- Water

BIBLIOGRAPHY

C .Sissoin 05/27/20, Medically reviewed by J. Kubala, MS, RD, Nutrition. *What is the average percentage of water in the human body?*

K.McGrane RS, RD. (2019).

https://www.medicalnewstoday.com/articles/what-percentage-of-the-human-body-is-water

https://tools.myfooddata.com/nutrient-ranking-tool/Water/Vegetables/Highest/Household/Common/No

https://www.healthline.com/nutrition/black-rice-benefits#_noHeaderPrefixedContent

https://vkool.com/benefits-of-butternut-squash/

www.ingramcontent.com/pod-product-compliance
Lightning Source LLC
Chambersburg PA
CBHW042055060526
44119CB00118B/321